THE PIG FARMER'S VETERINARY BOOK

CONTENTS

ILLUSTRATIONS

FOREWORD

by R. Braude, D.Sc., Ph.D., F.I.Biol.

THERE can be no better testimonial for a book than the publication of its tenth edition. On such an occasion, our first thought is to congratulate most heartily the author and the publishers on an outstanding achievement.

It is very gratifying that this popular guide for practical pig keepers is being continuously brought up-to-date by the author. He has certainly been watching carefully what has been happening around pigs and adding useful advice on day-to-day operations in the piggery.

Great progress has been made in pig production since the publication of the first edition, but at no time has the health aspect been more important than it is now. Healthy pigs grow faster, utilize their feed more efficiently, make management easier and the work in the piggery more congenial—all factors contributing to a profitable, satisfying and well worthwhile enterprise.

Throughout this book the author endeavours to educate on health matters and to guide on prevention of disease and of other difficulties in the piggery. Having done this effectively, he gives authoritative advice on what a pig keeper should do when ill-fate or mismanagement lands his animals in trouble.

R. Braude

Reading

AUTHOR'S PREFACE

TO THE FIRST EDITION

THE losses which the pig industry suffers today are far too heavy. These are due to a number of factors, not the least of which is our relative ignorance of the environmental conditions necessary for full health and maximum growth. What knowledge and experience we have appears to be possessed by all too few. Perhaps this book will help to remedy this defect to some extent.

It is not meant to replace the veterinary surgeon on the farm, as of course in the control of any disease, a proper diagnosis is the first essential. Clinical symptoms may be confusing and faulty treatment may be introduced if this is not correct, but an understanding of the possibilities regarding treatment should encourage help to be sought with greater confidence. Emphasis throughout the book, however, is upon the environmental conditions which play so vital a part in connection with keeping an animal so artificially reared as the pig usually is.

Many chance remarks by pigmen and farmers, together with the assistance of my veterinary colleagues, have proved invaluable in enabling me to compile this book and to all these, I would like to express my thanks.

NORMAN S. BARRON

Reading

AUTHOR'S PREFACE

TO THE EIGHTH EDITION

ONCE more it is pleasing to be able to report progress in the field of pig health, though the sudden arrival of SVD from a distant European source has certainly given us a shock and provided a reminder of our vulnerability. Whether this disease must be added to our list of permanent residents is cause for much debate. But with a more positive attitude to the dangers of swill as a distributing agent and a better knowledge of the vagiaries of the SVD virus, there is reason for optimism.

Set patterns of TGE are becoming clear and progress in vaccination techniques in this and *E. coli* scours is breaking fresh ground. The idea of surface cell immunity is well confirmed and applies to most surfaces such as the respiratory and mammary surfaces.

Behavioural studies are being vigorously pursued and suggest that the pig is not unlike the human in its anomalous and sometimes barbaric reaction to circumstances.

We have the tools to make the pig industry even more efficient than it is—if only more farmers would use them.

NORMAN S. BARRON

Reading

AUTHOR'S PREFACE

TO THE NINTH EDITION

THE continued popularity of a book on diseases might well make the pessimist put his money back in his pocket and throw up his hands in despair. But all is not lost. Considerable progress has been made in the reduction and control of many diseases. SVD has come and almost gone. It had the advantage of drawing attention to the appalling state of swill production and was the final justification, if any were needed (viz, foot and mouth, swine fever and Newcastle disease) to bring this process under strict control. We may well also see a reduction in salmonellosis.

The pattern of certain conditions has come into focus as a result of experience. TGE can be more easily recognised and controlled; the cause of swine dysentery (the spirochaete, *Treponema hyodysenteriae*) is now accepted, though some of the trigger mechanisms remain obscure. Nutrition is becoming steadily more sophisticated with its trace minerals, vitamins and growth promoters, not to mention appetisers for piglets such as apple juice and chocolate chips.

With changing systems of management in an endeavour to improve profitability, including that of concentration of stock, other problems arise—and always will. Rhinitis has now replaced enzootic pneumonia and 'stress' has become an interfering factor, if not a disease in its own right.

But we can take heart that interest and activity are evident in all fields—building, management and veterinary—which only serves to reaffirm the fact that wise management means better health and less disease.

NORMAN S. BARRON

Reading

AUTHOR'S PREFACE

TO THE TENTH EDITION

THIS is surely a time for celebration coinciding as it does with the twentieth anniversary of this book. It is hoped that to the many readers it has proved beneficial and to them my thanks are due. But change is endemic and the rapid expansion of the pig industry has brought with it a spectacular change in management methods, buildings, feeding and breeding, all of which have had, and will continue to have a major impact on health.

In this context, perhaps the concentration of stock has had the greatest influence affecting the individual behaviour of the pig and has moreover greatly increased the risks of the spread of disease. Management has barely kept up with this hazard, as a result of which we now have to combat swine dysentery, the pneumonias and rhinitis on a major scale—no easy task.

However, the need to ensure disease-free stock from the start, the greater understanding of environmental factors, the importance of stress and an improved therapeutic armoury give cause for optimism for the future.

NORMAN S. BARRON

Reading
February 1978

Chapter 1

PREVENTION THE BEST CURE

SUCCESS in pig-keeping depends largely upon proper management. Not only should the pigs be well housed and fed, but they should be kept in good health so that losses (and most of them can be prevented) are reduced to a minimum.

In the pages that follow we shall consider how this latter aim can be achieved.

COST OF DISEASE

The cost of disease in livestock is considerable. It is said to cost farmers in England and Wales alone over £1,000,000 every week.

Its cost to pig-keepers is very heavy. Not only is there the loss, very often, of the animals, but there is loss of time and labour and food that could be better spent on healthy stock. Statistical surveys have shown that of all the pigs born in this country, some 25 per cent die even before they are of weaning age. Eighty per cent of these losses occur during the first week, and losses are by no means rare in the later stages.

To lose one pig out of every four born is a severe handicap to profitable pig-keeping. Yet most of this loss can be prevented. It is a matter of good management.

Pigs, given access to what they need and would perhaps not

get under natural conditions, seldom fail to thrive. Such things as proper feeding, warmth and shelter are as essential to pigs as they are to us.

Attention to details is the mark of a good herdsman. Some farmers say that a herdsman is born and not made, but this is not true; the necessary details of management can be learnt by a keen man. There are special courses such as that run by the Agricultural Training Board which will help him in this direction.

To those who seek to make pig-keeping their livelihood or a profitable sideline, or to take charge of herds, this book is primarily addressed, and my first lesson is a simple one. It is that it is far better to prevent disease than to cure it.

This is where your skilled herdsman comes in. When feeding pigs his first thought is to see that all of them are eating heartily and none lying in a corner or under the straw. Coats should look clean and healthy and there should be no sign of lameness.

He is alert for the first indication of trouble. Measures taken now are likely to be the least costly and the most effective.

He will follow certain basic rules that are common to all successful pig-keepers. He will be careful neither to feed too much nor too little, both of which can cause loss. He won't forget the water. He will adjust his feeding to the different individual requirements of his pigs and he will watch for waste. In brief, he makes a thorough study of his job.

All these management details, followed as a matter of course by the skilled man, help to prevent the unthriftiness or low condition of health which leads inevitably to some form of disease and often to inexplicable deaths and serious loss in a herd.

The first lesson then is—look after your pigs carefully, study their requirements, keep an eye open for the first indication of illness, try to prevent trouble and, if it does come, call in your veterinary surgeon as soon as you can. In fact, why not have a 'health control' contract with him? Remember, a pig that is perfectly healthy one morning and eats its meal heartily can be dead by next morning through the sudden onset of disease.

Now for a word on another important subject that has a big effect on health. I refer to housing.

The pig is naturally an outdoor animal. It does well under free-range conditions. It is not so paradoxical therefore that pigs often do better under old, primitive conditions—conditions that might be described as "more natural"—than they do in many modern architectural palaces, which are cold and uncomfortable.

Housing plays an extremely important part in intensive pig management, affecting growth, health and economic prosperity. Indeed, bad housing can be a primary cause of ill-health and disease and under this heading must be included the completely automated system, which while it has many advantages, cuts off the pigman from his stock and makes inspection a rarity rather than a commonplace. Early signs of disease may thus be overlooked.

Depopulation of buildings from time to time is very essential to reduce disease build-up. All orifices should be closed and the premises gassed for 12–24 hours, or thoroughly cleaned down with hot soda solution followed by a disinfectant and left vacant for a week to dry out. This applies particularly to farrowing houses or units and to buildings to be used for imported stock.

RECORDS

Finally the advantages of keeping records as a means of enabling the trouble to be spotted before it builds up to a serious problem, cannot be over-emphasised; let your veterinary surgeon see these each time he comes.

There could be evidence of a fall in numbers born, reduced birth weights, a rise in the proportion born dead (under developed or fully grown) or mummies, splay-leg, no anus, hernias, etc.

Chapter 2

PIGS MUST BE COMFORTABLE

PIGS need to be warm and comfortable. These two fundamental needs must be met by the housing you use for pigs if your pig-keeping is to be successful. If you rear pigs in conditions that are unsatisfactory in these respects, you will run the risk of losses through disease.

Further, you will not be making the best use of feedingstuffs; the number of pounds (kg) of meat you will get for the pounds (kg) of food eaten will be fewer than if the pigs were in the right environment. In other words, the food conversion rate will be poor. An improvement of 0·1 in this respect is worth more in terms of food saved than any other improvement except one extra piglet at weaning.

The importance of proper conditions cannot be over-emphasised. Because pigs are naturally out-of-door animals, many people seem to think they like and need plenty of draughts, muck and mud.

This is not so. We now know, for example, that cold, damp conditions will encourage the onset of anaemia in young pigs and their subsequent death from the disease, even when they have been previously treated with iron as an anti-anaemia safeguard. On the other hand, pigs—fattening pigs in particular—can withstand, and in fact seem to prefer, a high humidity so long as the temperature is also high. Under all circumstances it is most important that the temperature is uniform and does not fluctuate appreciably.

Now this does not mean you have got to provide expensive and palatial accommodation for your pigs. Their housing can be cheap and even rough—provided that it is warm and dry where they rest and sleep.

Pigs in their natural wild state adjust themselves to their surroundings. From woodland undergrowth they build snug and rainproof farrowing nests and community dens. They keep them dry too. No dung or urine is passed in these shelters.

After passing through an arbitrary phase, the need for comfort (warmth, good ventilation, lack of draughts) is now fully realised and in general is reflected in good housing design using proper insulating materials and adequate slurry disposal systems. Heating systems, except in the farrowing house, are rare; in the fattening house it is sometimes forgotten that it is the pigs that keep the place warm. So ideally a house should be full to capacity.

MODERN FARROWING PEN

Today farrowing pens are single units, each with its own equipment (crate, water and food trough and side creeps) and often grouped in one heated building. The sow only needs a temperature of 60°F (16°C). The idea that a few bars across a corner, with a light above, provides a satisfactory creep area has, alas, contributed to much ill health and loss. Ground draughts are in fact encouraged by the heat in the corner, and the situation is made even worse for the piglets even if the main object of preventing crushing has been achieved.

I cannot lay too much stress on the importance of the creep being box-like in structure, with the lamps passing through the roof. A peep-hole may be provided if required, or the roof may be in the form of a lid. The way the pigs are lying will give you an immediate indication as to whether the creep is comfortable or not. If they are piled up on each other, seeking warmth from each other's bodies, then they are not at ease. If they are lying singly and spread out, conditions are obviously suitable to them.

TRY THIS TEST

To readers who are seriously prepared to tackle the job of seeing that their pig accommodation is warm enough, I suggest the purchase of a thermometer. One with a maximum and minimum setting is best; it will show how low the temperature falls during the night.

Try this in one of your pig-houses for a full 24 hours during a wintry spell. Suspend it from the roof of the house so that it hangs near, but not directly over, the sleeping section and just out of the animals' reach. Then read off the minimum temperature recorded during the period. Repeat the procedure in your other pig-houses; and try it again during a hot spell in summer with an eye to the maximum temperatures reached.

It is a good plan occasionally to visit your pigs in the early hours of the morning, and you will then be able to satisfy yourself that the conditions are comfortable.

I have a feeling that the results may surprise you, particularly the winter recordings, and especially when you compare them with the following temperatures that have been proved by research as the most suitable temperatures for proper health and growth:

For a sow and litter—80° F (27° C) in the creep.
For pigs from $3\frac{1}{2}$ to 7 score—62-65° F (17-18° C).
For pigs from $8\frac{1}{2}$ score upwards—60° F (16° C).

Where houses fail to give these conditions, and particularly if they have a tendency to dampness as well, the risk of ill-health and disease arising is considerable.

How then can the right conditions be most nearly obtained when building a pig-house or converting an existing farm building for pigs?

First, siting a new building. It is well to take advantage of any natural shelter, particularly from the north and east winds.

Secondly, floors. In some circumstances wire mesh may replace concrete but when the latter is used, especially for adults, the anti-slip finish of the surface must be considered. Much damage is done to feet and limbs if this is overlooked. (See also under Biotin, page 91).

Something should be done to warm concrete up. Electricity is generally too expensive. An air space below the surface is the best means. This can be obtained by using land tiles, air-bricks, bottles or other materials below the surface concrete.

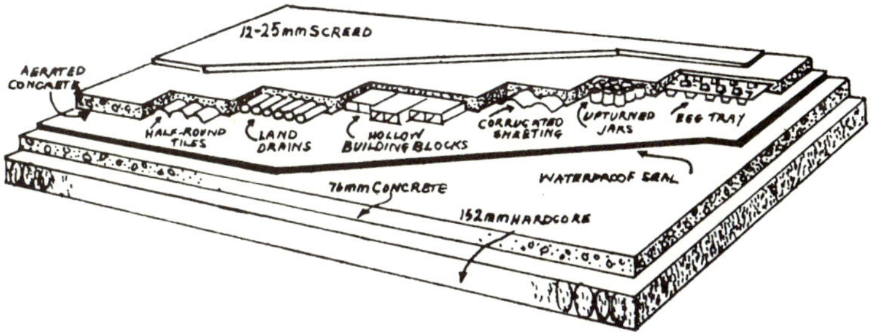

Cheap and effective floor insulation.

Where you have an existing concrete floor that is not insulated for warmth and you wish to avoid relaying it, you should consider providing a raised section that can be insulated from the main floor.

One way of doing this is to lay a sheet of corrugated asbestos or polystyrene on the existing concrete and then cover this with another two or three inches (50-75 mm) of concrete. Alternatively, a movable wooden floor on 2-in (50 mm) joists can be provided, but this may sometimes be rather unsatisfactory from the point of view of hygiene for wood does not stand up well to the action of urine. Such floors are, however, quite satisfactory for sows and litters provided that room is allowed for exercise and dunging.

With floor feeding, the feeding and sleeping area is the same. If troughs are used, this decides the number of pigs per unit. Eight inches (200 mm) is allowed and all pigs must be able to feed together.

One further point arises in connection with floor construction. That is drainage for urine.

Each individual pen in a community house should drain directly into a common channel *outside* the building, rather than through another pen. When a drainage system of this kind cannot be provided and where pigs have to use a corner of their pen for urinating, ample straw bedding must be given to avoid setting up cold, damp conditions. Further, good ventilation—but not a draught—is essential to carry off ammonia fumes.

In an effort to simplify and reduce labour costs of dung disposal, the system of liquid dung disposal is now common. The dung, if liquid enough, is swept down to and through the slats over the take-away channel, or the dunging passage is covered with slats so that the excreta falls directly, or is trodden through, into the underground channel below. The liquid effluent is then removed by appropriate means and spread on fields or arable land. Alternatively, where the dung is semi-solid it can be stacked and made into good compost by mixing with old straw in the close vicinity of the piggery.

Care must be taken to ensure the proper siting of the slats. These must be strong enough to withstand the weight of the heaviest pigs and yet sufficiently wide apart to allow the passage of the excreta without catching the pigs' feet. So far concrete has proved better than wire or timber. Pigs have been known to fall through broken slats and drown. The gases from slurry are also poisonous in high concentration to both pigs and man.

MATERIALS TO USE

Now with regard to the materials used for pig-house construction.

Here the essential requirement from a veterinary point of view is to choose one which is not greatly susceptible to temperature fluctuation. In this respect the insulating value is of extreme importance, and such materials as bonded resin sheets are very satisfactory, but there are many excellent materials available from which the architect or farmer may choose.

Whichever material you use, a cavity wall—*i.e.* a double wall with an air space between—will improve matters. The inner wall need not be of the same material as the outer wall. Indeed, with metal buildings—*e.g.* nissen huts—this would be most inadvisable. These should be lined above the supporting walls with sheets of some sort of insulating material. In a large hut, or one that is not adequately warmed by the pigs within, a false roof may be necessary.

INSULATING THE ROOF

Corrugated iron or asbestos sheeting are widely used because they are cheap and easy to work with. However, as their insulating qualities are poor, resulting in heavy condensation, a false roof should be fixed 4-5 ft (1·2 to 1·5 m) above the pigs and extend 5-6 ft (1·5 to 1·8 m) out from the rear wall over the resting area. It should be light and so constructed that it can be removed and replaced at intervals. Such a roof can be simply made by using 1 in (25 mm) wire-netting supporting a 3-4 in (75-100 mm) layer of straw. There are all sorts of alternatives, such as hurdles, laths of wood, which can be covered with loose straw or upon which straw bales may be placed. Sisalkraft laid on the wire-netting will prevent the straw from being pulled through by the pigs. Paper bags may also be used.

Of course, it is far better to line corrugated or asbestos sheeting with fibreboard or some suitable material, always remembering to seal the joints appropriately. If the roof is too high a light, false roof covering the whole area should be fitted.

VENTILATION

Now, having discussed every possible way to ensure that a building is warm in winter, it becomes necessary to see that it gets a proper supply of fresh air, rather than draughts.

For a natural system of ventilation the square box-shaft or chimney has proved satisfactory in many piggeries. For example, in a Harper Adams piggery one outlet in the roof and three inlets placed in the walls just above pig height would be sufficient for a pair of pens.

However, more and more pig-keepers are using extraction ventilation fans. This system ensures that an adequate amount of air passes through the building. Generally speaking, air

VENTILATION CONTROL

1. Natural ventilation

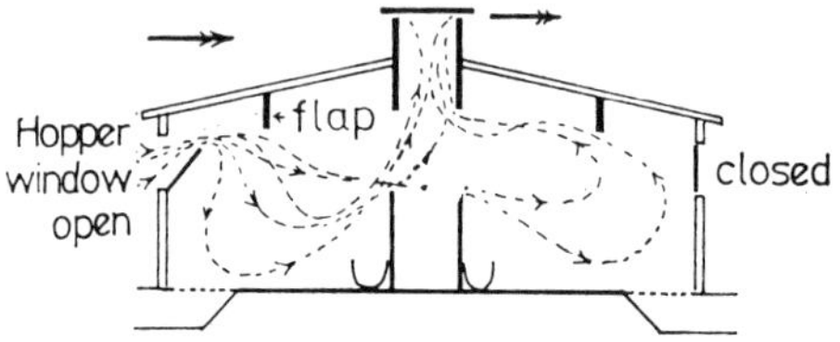

2. Natural ventilation

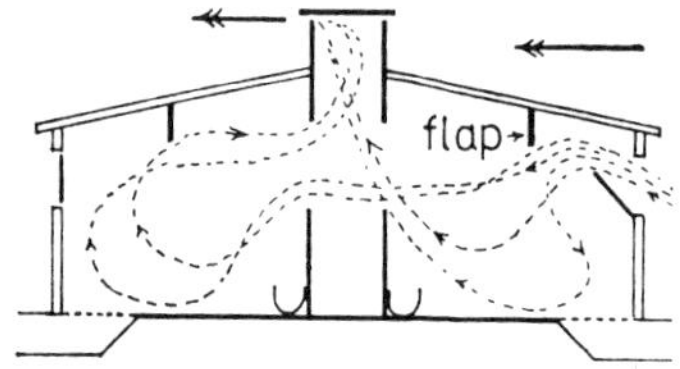

Natural ventilation depends on wind movement. Hopper windows open on windward side, while flaps project air downwards.

3. Lateral suction fans

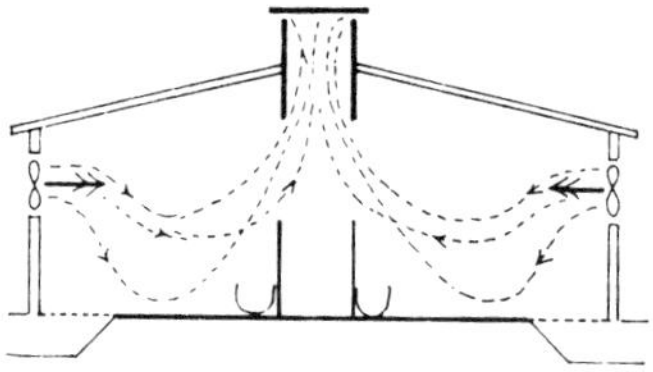

4. Lateral extraction fans

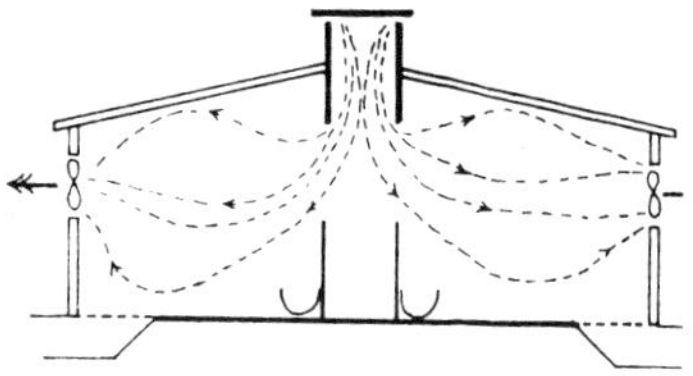

5. Vertical suction fan

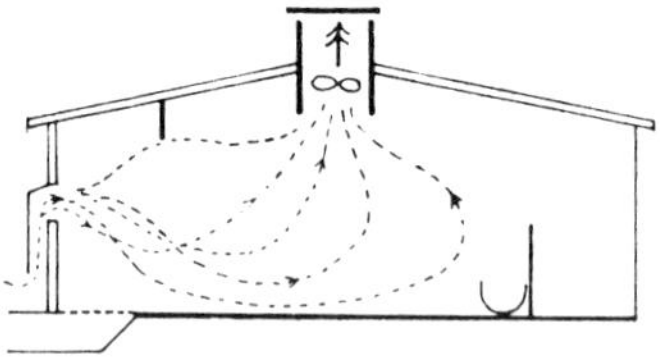

6. Vertical injection fan

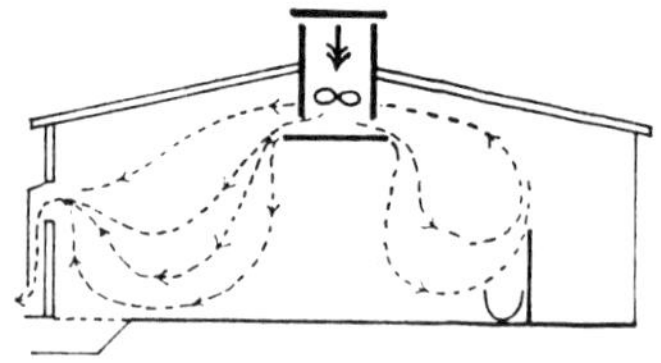

Air should be changed frequently, but never so fast that movement is noticeable. Blow air gently on to the pigs first, and lastly over the dunging area before elimination from building.

inlets of about 4-6 sq in (26-39 cm^2) per pig should be evenly spaced round the walls (often one grating per pair of pens is satisfactory). The extract shafts should be about 18 in (116 cm^2) square; usually two per building are sufficient, spaced at about one-third in from each gable end. To avoid occasional stagnation, electrically-driven extraction fans could be installed in the shafts. The important point to observe is that the cold air should not fall on the pigs' backs, nor should the foul air be extracted over them.

It is best to adhere to exact standards which maintain a uniform temperature, be it low or high. A humid atmosphere would seem to be more beneficial than one that is exceedingly dry. The former, especially when excessive, appears to be soothing to the respiratory tract, and the reported reduction in pneumonia infections and coughing in general may well be due to the greater tendency for the sedimentation of particles, swollen by the dampness in the atmosphere, to carry bacteria down, as compared with a rapidly-moving dry and dusty environment. Coughing is certainly more common under the latter conditions.

The most frequent cause of a draught is the roof of a building being too high. This creates a down-draught and allows too great a volume of air per pig. Pigs want the roof well down, as low as is compatible with ease of working when cleaning out. They will, to some extent, keep the building warm with their own body heat. But remember that this is only possible, especially in the winter time when the building is full, or nearly full, of pigs.

I would regard 6 ft (1·8 m) at the eaves, rising to 8 ft (2·4 m) at the ridge, as satisfactory where it is necessary for a person to enter and work in a building for mucking-out purposes. Where an open dunging yard is provided, roofs can be lower than this with advantage.

Light is not important for fattening pigs, in fact there appear to be advantages in keeping them in the dark. A light dunging passage or yard will, however, attract the pigs and prevent them from soiling their bedding.

A final point on permanent houses concerns the use of a common dunging passage and an open drainage channel within the building.

This system is not a good thing from a veterinary point of view. Disease germs can be passed in the dung or urine, and during the process of sweeping the manure right down the length of the passage, infection can be spread to pigs in other pens, which is all important when dealing with salmonellosis, vibrionic dysentery, and TGE. A channel under slats is, however, a good thing.

SWEAT BOXES

In this system there is no planned ventilation so that humidity builds up to saturation point and moisture collects on the roof and walls, and drips down on to the floor. An essential feature of the process, however, is the maintenance of a uniform temperature of 78-85° F (25-29° C). There must be sufficient pigs in the pen to maintain this level—and the temperature *must* be maintained. A sudden fall in temperature will chill the pigs and result in a breakdown of the whole system.

Light is not necessary for growth so there are no windows. This avoids one unnecessary stress factor. Pigs appear to be completely relaxed and lying contentedly against each other between meals. Animals suffering from pneumonia seem to find conditions relaxing and coughing is very rare (see droplet infection under enzootic pneumonia, page 124).

It cannot be denied that the sweat-box system is aesthetically most unattractive, but it is also true that many pigs housed under more orthodox methods are frequently to be found under conditions which are atrocious and even inhuman. If we admit that restriction of exercise is necessary in the latter stages of growth then there is nothing basically wrong with the sweat-box system.

FLOOR SPACE

Dealing with the floor space, the normal recommendation is 80 sq ft (7·4 m^2) per sow and litter. Thus an area of about 10 ft by 8 ft (3 m by 2·5 m) is satisfactory for a farrowing pen, but provision should be made for a dunging, feeding and exercising area.

It is best to reduce floor space to a minimum in the fattening pen; for a fully-grown pig allow about 5 sq ft (0·46 m^2) for the sleeping quarters and 6 sq ft (0·56 m^2) for the yard or dunging area.

Now a word about the rough temporary types of outdoor shelter, many of which are proving highly satisfactory.

Some of these improvised shelters are good. One of the best I have seen consisted simply of several curved sheets of metal from an Anderson shelter laid on the ground.

With turves laid against both edges and one end blocked with straw, this makes an almost perfect shelter for little pigs. It would, however, be over-warm in fierce sun; a covering of loose straw would help in this respect.

Shelters made of straw bales with roughly thatched roofs are also good. But they have the big disadvantage that they are not readily movable. This is essential for outdoor housing, particularly on heavy and wet land; for if pigs have to go through mud to get into and out of their shelter, they will quickly make their bedding damp, thus bringing about the very conditions I have been campaigning against in this chapter.

But a simple, more portable system, now very popular, involves the use of huts made of arches of corrugated iron galvanised sheets, one end of which is blocked off by wooden boards or bales of straw, the other end being open or, if necessary protected by straw bales. These huts can be used for all purposes all the year round, but when used for farrowing a front board is desirable for the first week after farrowing to prevent piglets from straying and to discourage invaders from stealing a drink. A simple wooden creep constructed parallel to the side will keep the food dry and enable piglets to eat from troughs not accessible to the sow.

Some farmers prefer properly constructed wooden huts on skids. These can be used folded over the ground and brought in on to hard ground or concrete when weather conditions are bad or the system demands it.

There is a big health advantage in keeping pigs out-of-doors; it is well to make most of this by seeing that they have good accommodation which will give them adequate protection from the weather when they need it.

CONVERTING COVERED YARDS

Where covered yards (such as have been used for winter bullock fattening in the past) are used for keeping pigs, a big problem arises. These yards are often far too airy for pigs in winter and as they are frequently roofed with metal, they are over-hot in summer.

Only an expensive conversion will make a large yard really suitable for pigs. Nevertheless it is possible to reduce its disadvantages a little by some inexpensive measures.

Walls of straw bales to block up open ends and possibly to sub-divide the yard are worth considering. So are double wire-netting walls packed with straw.

But even with these added means of protection, I think it desirable to see that pigs in yards always have an abundance of loose straw in which they can snuggle for warmth, or a roofed-over shelter along one side. Weaners from 8-12 weeks benefit especially if allowed to exercise in straw-yards.

The use of sowstalls is already an innovation and has many attractions, but before such equipment is installed the design should be carefully studied. The length and width of the stalls, and the nature of the slats, are very important.

All this, of course, boils down to studying the principal needs of pig housing in whatever method of pig-keeping you wish to follow. You cannot make a bigger mistake than neglect to provide warm and comfortable accommodation, with satisfactory ventilation but without draught.

If you will do this, you will be going a long way to preventing disease in pigs.

Chapter 3

GENERAL SIGNS OF HEALTH AND DISEASE

BEFORE getting down to the actual job of dealing with ill-health when it arises, I want to discuss another factor in disease control. This is the important matter of recognising when a pig is "off colour".

The onset of disease in a pig can be sudden; its development can be quick. An animal may be apparently normal one day and may seem to eat heartily; yet, within 24 hours it can be dead from some infection or disorder.

Now if a pig farmer or herdsman wants to prevent these sudden losses, he must be quick, too. He must be quick to recognise the slightest departure from normal—the first indication of trouble—and he must be quick to apply the appropriate remedy or get someone else to do so.

POINTS TO LOOK FOR

So you see how important it is to be able to spot an ailing pig before anything is seriously wrong.

To be skilled in this needs long experience. Nevertheless the skill can be developed by close observation. These are the points that should be studied:

General Attitude of Animal: In health this should reflect vigour and well-being. There should be an alert look, the ears pricked (except, of course, in the case of lop-eared pigs), the tail curled. The snout should be moist and shining, the ears warm to the touch.

The mucous membrane (observed inside lower eyelid, by parting lips of vulva or by examining gums) should be salmon pink. It may be very deep pink or even red in feverish conditions or extremely pale in cases of collapse or loss of blood. In cases of jaundice it is yellow.

In contrast with these signs of health, an ailing pig will have a general appearance of dullness. There will be a lack of bloom, the coat will lose its shine, have a staring appearance and may be wrinkled and greasy. The tail generally loses its curl and droops, and the ears are cold.

WATCH THE SKIN

Skin Coloration: Pigs often show exaggerated skin colorations which are not diagnostic of disease.

These may be a diffuse pink or a deep purple. They may be confined to a limited area, such as the throat and ears, or affect the skin over a large area. The skin may be as deeply coloured when the pig is constipated as when it is suffering from a serious disease such as swine fever.

The "diamondings" seen in erysipelas are characteristic; in cases of acute swine fever there may be many haemorrhages under the skin, and the rashes associated with mange, parakeratosis, pityriasis, ringworm and pig pox, help to establish a diagnosis. The skin, however, should not be wrinkled, scurfy or greasy with scrabs or irregular patches of inflammation and there should be no lice present—although these do often occur even on thriving pigs. A paper-white or faintly yellowish skin is often present in anaemia in young pigs.

A gross thickening of the skin may be associated with erysipelas, and when dark in colour and scaly is often described as "elephant skin" and is characteristic of the so-called non-specific skin rash (parakeratosis). If red and "pimply" and limited in distribution, and irritation is present, the existence of mange parasites is to be suspected.

A normal skin is quite white or faintly pink and shiny,

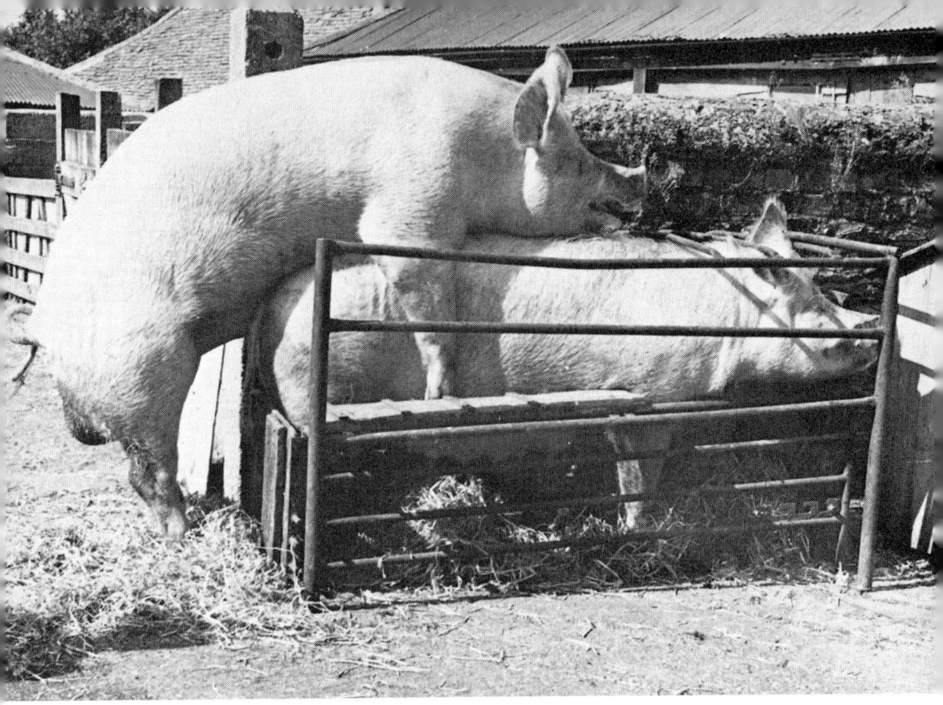

This service crate restrains the sow and takes the boar's weight off her during mating.

Pregnancy can be diagnosed within 30 days of service by snipping off a tiny piece of the sow's vagina and examining it under a microscope.

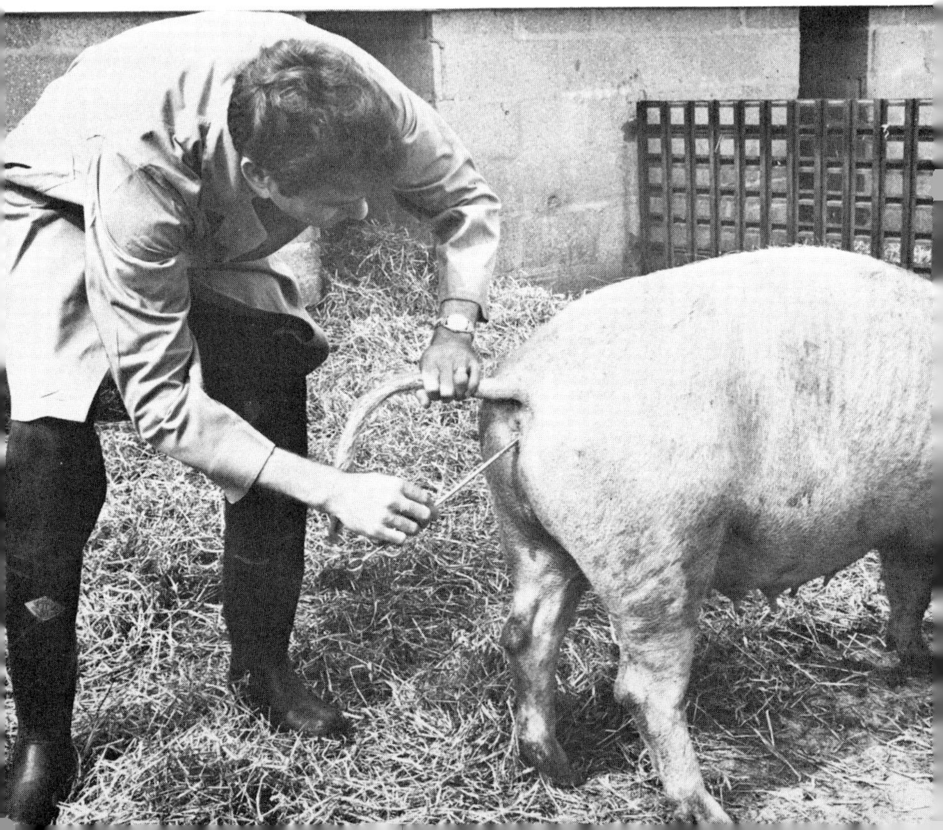

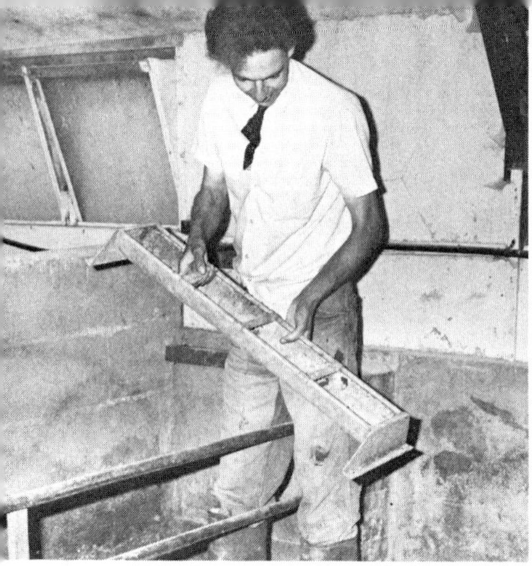

When cleaning pens, start by clearing out all equipment and removable fittings.

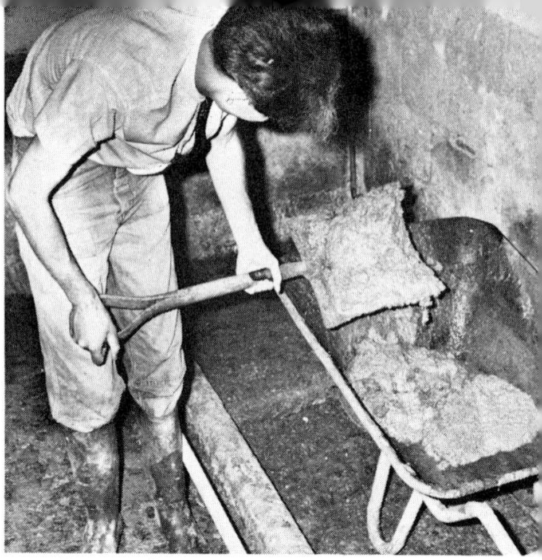

Scrape off muck and remove from pen.

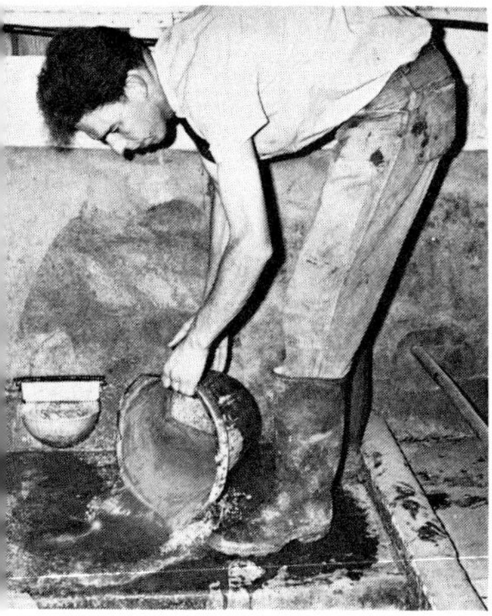

Flood floor with soda solution and brush vigorously.

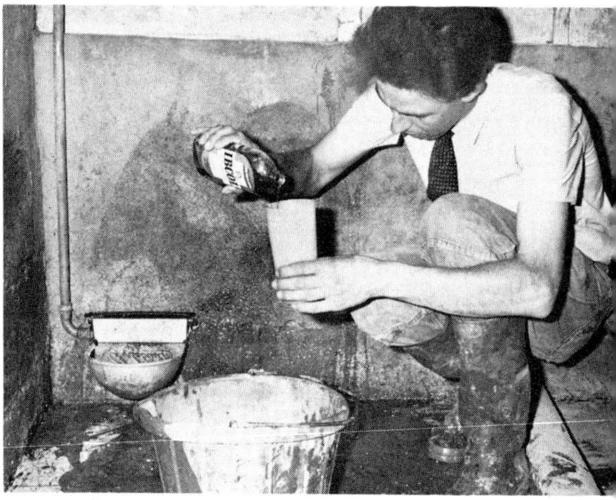

Use a plastic measuring jar to measure correct amount of disinfectant.

Four second spray, add 4 parts tricthylene glycol (anti-freeze solution) to each 6 parts of concentrated disinfectant.

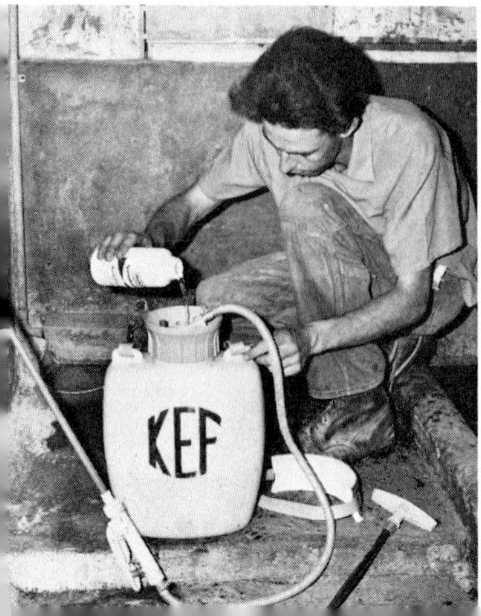

Finally—fumigation. Mix 3 parts liquid formalin with 2 parts potassium permanganate in a flat dish. To avoid scalding splashes, always put potassium permanganate in first.

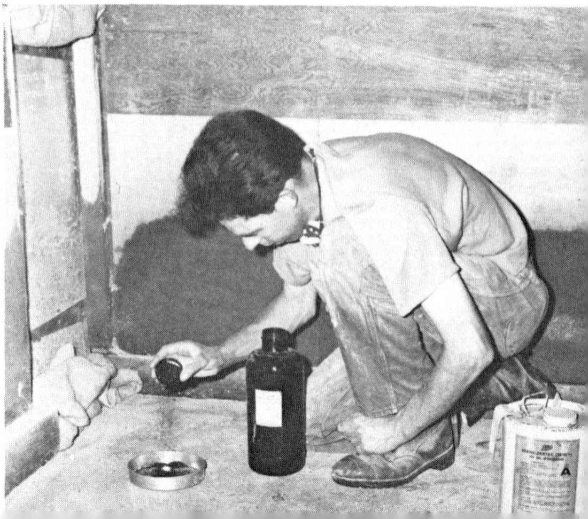

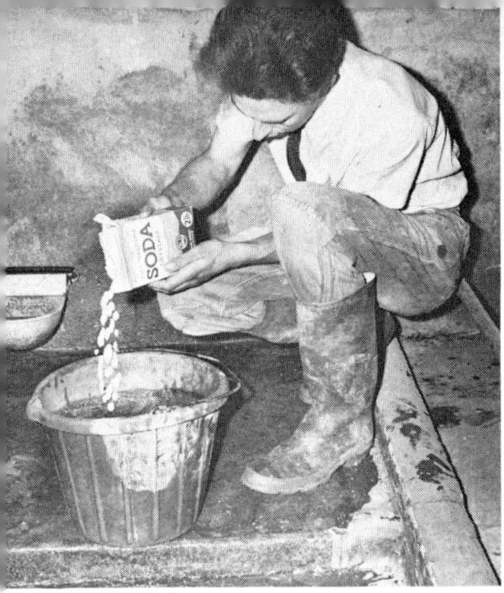

Vashing soda (454 g per 11.5 litres of hot
ater) removes dirt from walls and floors
nd kills most germs.

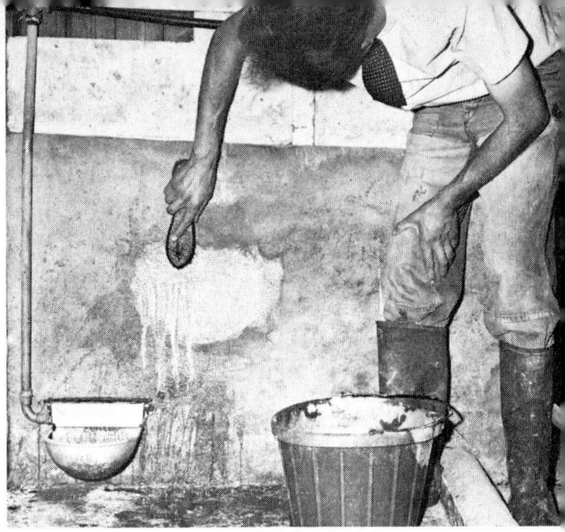

Scrub walls to pen-division height.

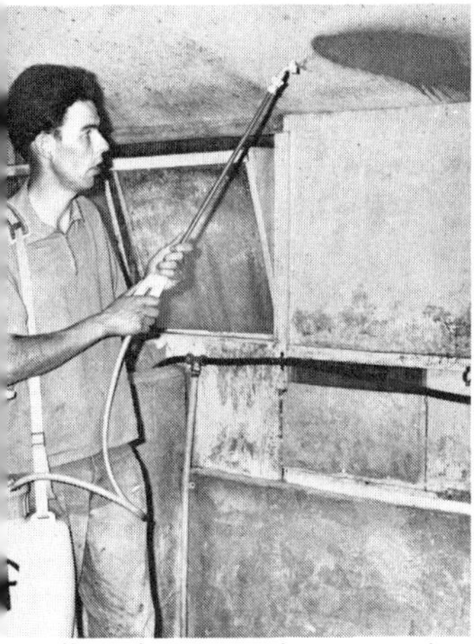

y walls, ceiling & pen divisions with
fectant using a fine-mist nozzle.

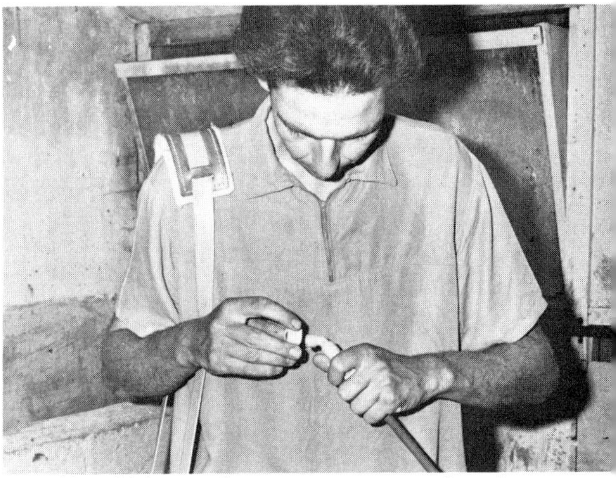

After 24 hours, change to a coarse nozzle and spray again.

ow 500 ml of formalin for each 900 m² of air space. Wear
nask to avoid inhaling fumigant gas. Leave building sealed
24 hours.

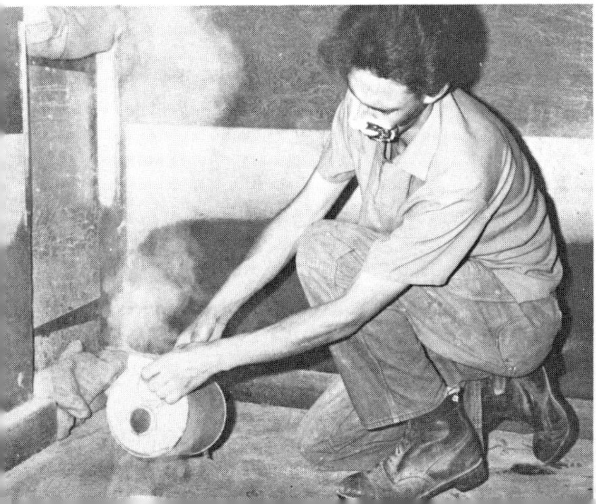

Soak troughs in soda solution for 24 hours. Then pressure-hose off dirt and dip in disinfectant.

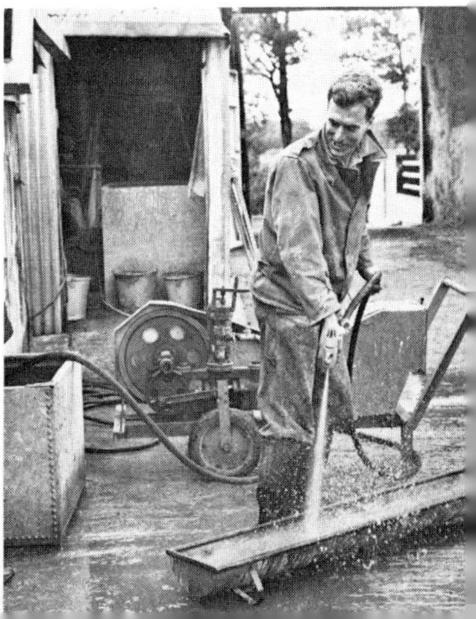

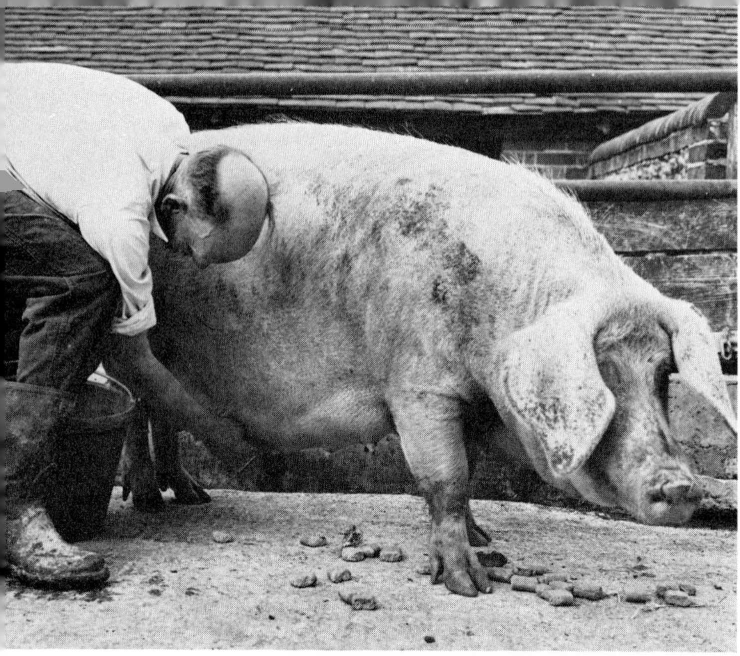

Wash sow's udde
before farrowing t
remove dirt and ad
hering worm eggs.

Also wash around her backside. Use warm water containing a detergent, then rinse with mild antiseptic solution.

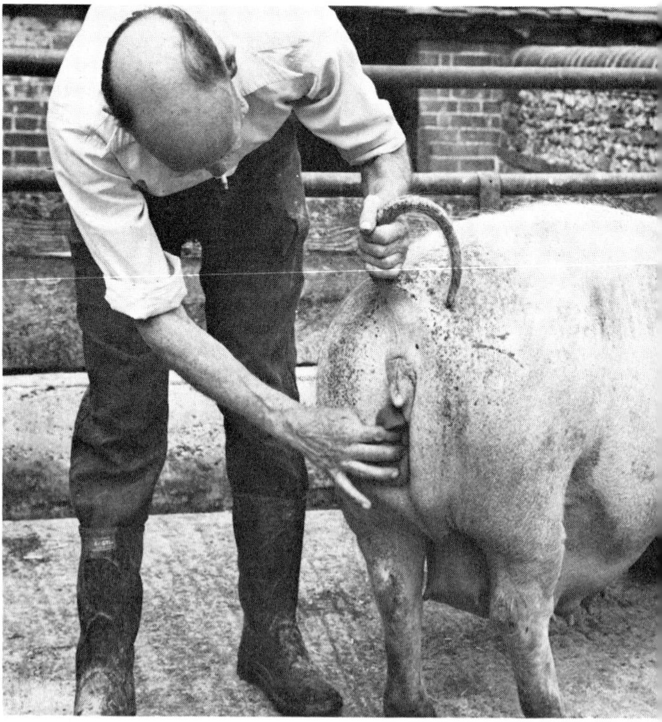

especially over the back. The latter feature can be observed even in black pigs.

NOT EATING

Appetite: This should be keen. If a pig does not come forward to eat at feeding time, it must be ailing.

But just a word of warning here. Although lack of appetite is one of the surest signs of trouble in the pig, it must not be taken as the only sign worth watching for. A pig may come forward and eat heartily even though it is in the early stages of some disorder.

If there is a tendency to lick woodwork or metal objects, this does not necessarily mean there is a nutritional deficiency though one could suspect a shortage of salt. Straw eating, for instance, may be purely due to boredom but it may, on the other hand, indicate an unsatisfied appetite, in so far as bulk is concerned. But do not rely upon variation in appetite alone, watch other points as well. Chewing stones can be associated with the presence of bowel worms.

Bodily Functions: Dung should be firm and formed roughly into large pellets with a slightly fibrous texture in the case of adults. It should not be too stringy, and a coating of mucus or blood is a bad sign.

In the sickening pig a light-coloured watery scour suggests anaemia, but in older pigs it may indicate swine fever or erysipelas. The dung may be hard and dark-coloured—often as a result of eating coal, cinders, acorns, or due to high level of copper in the diet—and may be very firm indeed in some cases of swine fever. Coarsely-ground meal is to be recommended, although if it is too coarse the particles may pass through the bowels undigested.

Blood in the droppings of store pigs suggests swine dysentery and a fluid scour is caused by worms or feverish conditions such as erysipelas or swine fever.

Urine should be anything from a pale yellow to a deep straw colour, but without any blood or abnormal coloration. It should be passed freely and without any sign of pain or discomfort. If blood pigment is present, this may be due to a diseased kidney, perhaps of bacterial origin (*C. suis*); if whole blood it may be due to direct injury of the bladder and/or urinary tract. Sows or gilts, however, may pass blood after being served by a too vigorous boar.

PULSE AND TEMPERATURE

Breathing should not be too heavy or erratic and it should be noiseless. Respirations (a rise and fall of the flanks counts as one complete respiration) should be at the rate of from 20 to 30 per minute in mature animals, but somewhat more rapid in young pigs.

The pulse rate (*i.e.* the heart beat) should be taken with the fingertips at the centre of the inside of the hind leg just below the level of the knee-cap (stifle). It should be within the range of 55 to 75 per minute.

The temperature (taken per rectum) should not be less than 101·2°F (38°C) and not more than 102·5°F (39°C). In the young pig after exercise this may rise naturally to 104°F (40°C) for a short time.

Respiration, pulse and temperature are all somewhat higher in early life and somewhat less in older animals. They can also be influenced by temperature of surroundings. Further, pulse and respiration will fluctuate spontaneously in response to excitement or shock—including the presence of a stranger.

These, then, are the points to look for in trying to get an early indication of disease.

Some of them—general appetite, condition of skin, respiration "beats" and appetite—can be observed without handling the animal. Others, like body temperature and colour of mucous membranes, cannot be ascertained without restraining the animal in some way.

Further, if the symptoms suggest an ailing condition, treatment needs to be given and that, too, frequently involves having the animal under control. But when something makes you suspect trouble in an animal, first watch it carefully without disturbing it in any way.

If it is resting, take the opportunity of counting its respirations. There won't be much value in a count taken after the pig has been chased around to try and capture it for more detailed examination.

While the pig is resting, you can also take stock of its general appearance and condition.

A more detailed examination involves some degree of control. How you can get that depends partly on the age of the pig concerned and partly on how friendly you (or the person who regularly handles your pigs) are with them. The secret in all cases is patience.

HANDLING PIGS

A few hints on the way to handle pigs and to give medicines, etc, will not come amiss at this stage. Let us go through the procedure step by step.

When dealing with fattening pigs, I find the best plan is to get them penned in a corner of the sty. A wooden door, light gate or hurdle or anything that makes a good barrier will do.

Having got them penned let them settle down. This they will readily do in a few minutes, usually obliging to such an extent that their heads are all pointing away from you, thus making the taking of temperatures per rectum an easy task; it also makes

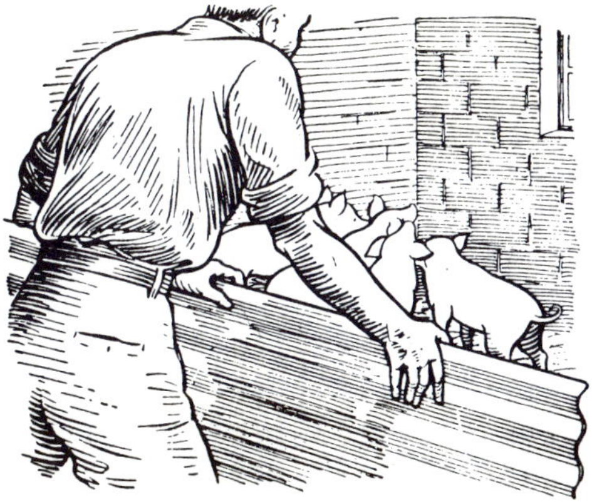

If you wish to handle young pigs, pen them in a corner with a sheet of galvanised iron or some other portable barrier.

it easier for the veterinary surgeon to give an intramuscular injection!

But whatever examination is being made or whatever treatment is being given to a litter penned like this, each animal should be marked with a paint stick after attention. Otherwise, because of re-shufflings, which are almost certain to occur, you may well do some animals more than once and some not at all. If the pigs are small enough they can be lifted out of the pen as soon as they have been treated.

WHEN ASSISTANCE IS NEEDED

Of course, baby pigs and growing pigs may have to be handled individually. So, an assistant is required for the job. He should hold the animal's ears, and the operator should hold the tail—thus leaving himself a free working hand.

Young pigs usually protest at this treatment. But again a little patience works wonders. Just hold on for a moment or two and the animal will invariably settle down and remain quiet for subsequent treatment.

Sows are usually quite amenable to examination and treatment, especially on farms where they are accustomed to a friendly word and a reassuring back-scratch.

Often a sow will stand while her temperature is taken if the farmer or herdsman scratches her back or tickles her belly. Injections can frequently be given without any further restraint being necessary.

But with strong store pigs, and especially with boars, it is usually necessary to take special steps to control them, although an attempt can first be made to force the animal against a wall or in a corner with some portable barrier.

If this doesn't succeed, resort will have to be made to slipping a running noose over the upper jaw and pulling it firmly backwards until the rope comes to rest behind the tushes. Then it can be tightened and the pig will be well under control.

It is usually necessary to approach the animal from behind to apply the rope.

When the rope is in place and tightened it can be securely

fastened to a gate-post or other convenient object that will withstand the strain. Where the animal has a nose ring, then a second rope can be slipped through it and secured to the same post or held by an assistant.

Another method is to use a running loop fixed on a metal rod which can be slipped over the upper jaw.

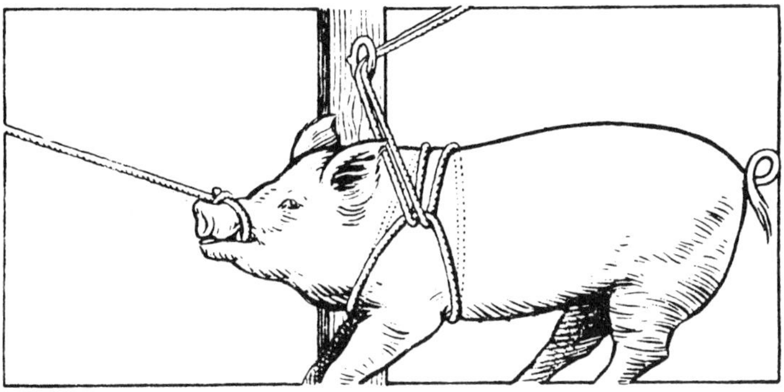

Method of restraining a pig when a simple running noose over upper jaw is inadequate.

Secured by either of these methods, the pig will usually lie back on the rope and is thus available for attention.

IN EXTREME CASES

But extreme cases do arise in which even this form of restraint is inadequate. For these I recommend, in addition to the rope around the upper jaw, a double rope passed round the body at the shoulders (one strand on either side of the front legs) with the two free ends passed through the loop, pulled tight and then slipped through a ring fastened to a stout post. The ring should be about 2-3 in (50-75 mm) above the pig's head (see sketch above).

With this form of control the pig is compelled to submit to whatever treatment you need to give.

A very effective alternative to the above methods is provided by the crate shown on page 39.

Because a pig usually fights against restraint it is better to avoid giving medicines in liquid form wherever possible. In the struggle that invariably takes place, there is a considerable risk that liquid may go into the lungs and cause pneumonia. This is most likely when the drench contains oil.

Where there is no alternative to liquids, a wooden mouth-gag with a hole in the middle is a useful instrument. Medicine can then be poured down a funnel to which is attached a stout piece of hose, the other end of which is inserted through the hole in the gag into the back of the mouth.

If this gadget is not available, the old-fashioned boot-with-a-hole-in-the-toe device may do the trick. The toepiece should be

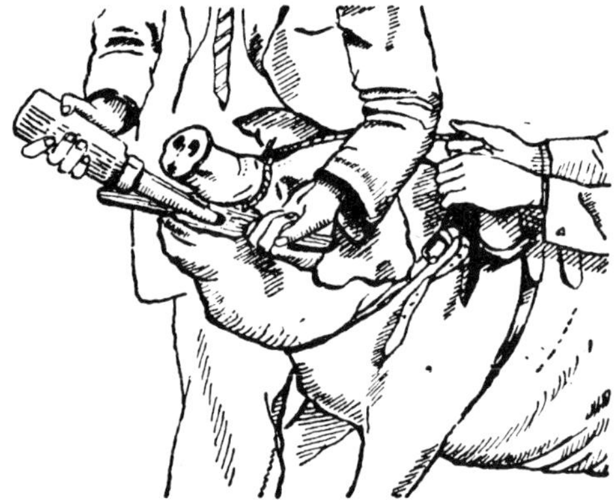

It is best to avoid giving medicines in liquid form —the liquid may get into the lungs—but when this is unavoidable, a wooden mouth gag is quite effective, and a bottle to which is fitted an old milking-machine liner.

inserted firmly into the mouth before the medicine is poured through the boot.

WHEN GIVING POWDERS

Powders and substances which will dissolve in water can, of course, be mixed with food. For this purpose it is often better to put the pigs on half rations for one meal before the doctored meal is given. This will ensure that it is all eaten.

At the same time a necessary precaution is to see that all the pigs in a pen (and there should not be too many) are of about

HANDY RINGING CRATE

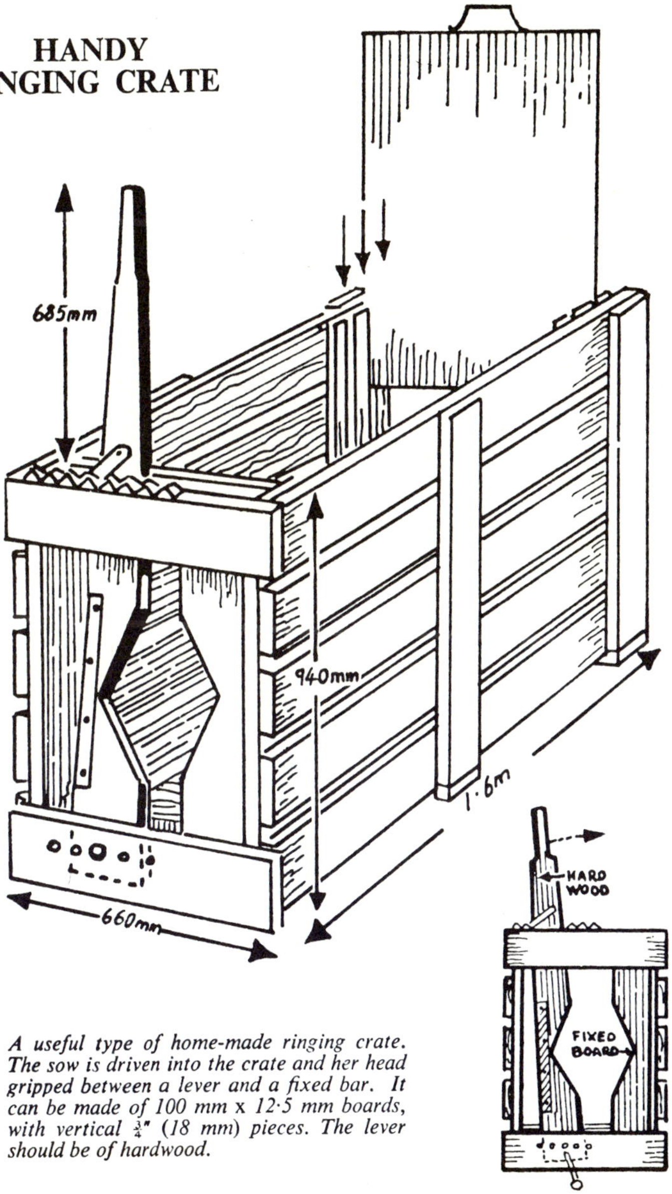

A useful type of home-made ringing crate. The sow is driven into the crate and her head gripped between a lever and a fixed bar. It can be made of 100 mm x 12·5 mm boards, with vertical ¾" (18 mm) pieces. The lever should be of hardwood.

equal size and weight, otherwise there is the risk that the stronger ones will eat more than their share of the food and, consequently, of the medicine.

For the same reason a nervous pig should not be included in a pen of pigs that "boss" it; it should be isolated temporarily.

Yet another form of offering a medicament is an electuary —a paste with a basis of treacle and flour containing the necessary "dope". This paste is usually scraped on to the teeth with a wooden spatula or the back of a wooden spoon.

VACCINES AND SERA

Apart from giving pills, powders and medicines, the treatment of disease nowadays involves the use of biological preparations such as vaccines and sera. The latter, as the name indicates, is the serum of an animal which has been either artificially or naturally protected against the disease for which it is being used.

For instance, swine erysipelas serum is prepared by giving horses a series of injections of the erysipelas germ. The protective antibodies produced in the horse's serum are conveyed to the blood of the pig at the time of injection. This method produces passive immunity which is generally short-lived. It will, however, give the animal immediate protection which declines by degrees over the following weeks as the antibodies become destroyed.

On the other hand, the practice of vaccination involves the injection of a material which will stimulate the injected animal to produce its own protective antibodies. Whilst it takes several weeks, as a rule, to build up a high degree of protection, the immunity so produced may last for many months. For instance, vaccination against swine erysipelas gives protection for about a year.

Injections may be given intravaneously, which means directly into the blood supply; subcutaneously, which means under the skin; or intramuscularly, deep into the muscle tissue.

The intramuscular injections are perhaps the most commonly used today. The needle of the syringe is inserted quickly, deeply into the muscle tissue. If it is possible to turn the animal on its back, then you can hold the hind legs with one hand and insert the needle of the syringe deep into the thick part of the leg by the hock.

If the pig is a large one, inject deeply behind the shoulder, inserting the needle in this case at an angle pointing forwards. The buttock, however, is the site of choice. Occasionally, injections are given subcutaneously behind the ear, but avoid getting into the pad of fat which lies there.

For those who wish to do their own injections several syringes should be secured. It would be useful to possess 2 c.c., 5 c.c. and 10 c.c. capacity syringes, either of the glass and metal record type of construction or of the expendable polythene type. The bore of the needle should increase with the size of the syringe and the length be from 1 inch to 1½ inches (25 mm to 37·5 mm).

In order to avoid damage or abscess formation the site of the injection should first be wiped clean with cotton wool soaked in methylated spirits. Have the animal firmly restrained and keep the syringe straight to avoid breaking the needle.

Another method of administering drugs—liquids, or powders dissolved in liquids—is by the mouth (orally) using the methods already described, and one must not forget the simple way of mixing with the food. Many medicinal agents, e.g. for treatment of worms, or growth promoters, are applied in this way.

Chapter 4

YOUR FIRST AIM—LARGE AND HEALTHY LITTERS

YOUR pig-keeping will not be profitable unless your sows produce large and healthy litters. So we will first tackle disease control and the prevention of losses during the cycle of reproduction.

It pays handsomely to start with healthy stock. Today there is a good choice of certified healthy accredited herds and you can also buy from MD established herds, which is your best bet. Put clean stock on to clean premises.

If you are selecting from your own breeding stock, select from sows that have had four litters. These will have a fair degree of immunity against most common conditions—scours, TGE, rhinitis, EP—and will hand on some in their colostrum. Avoid buying in in-pig animals if possible, but in any case isolate any imports for at least 14 days and preferably more. Breeding stock should be run on old litter to enable them to pick up the resident infective agents and so build up immunity. Cull your own stock hard.

OPEN-AIR LIFE

It pays to give your gilts and sows an open-air life as far as possible. They will benefit nutritionally by being turned out to grass, aftermath, potatoes, etc, but too much emphasis should not be laid upon the nutritional value of these crops. Pigs should, at the same time, receive rations containing high-grade animal protein and an adequate supply of minerals and vitamins in meal or nut form. The system of individual feeding which is increasing in popularity is extremely valuable and preferable if good healthy litters are to be achieved.

Bullying is so common among groups of in-pig gilts or dry sows that some do not get their full quota of food and so are not able to give of their best. They are likely to produce poor-quality litters, low in weight, and even containing a number of dead pigs.

RECOMMENDED FEEDING SYSTEM

Your aim should be to obtain a litter of not less than 12 weighing not less than 3 lb (1·4 kg) each at birth. By securing good birth-weights the survival rate is likely to be high, enabling freshly-born piglets to move more readily and avoid crushing. They will suckle more freely and be able to build up their resistance to disease quickly.

To secure a satisfactory number of piglets, flushing of the sow is an advantage where this is possible, but it depends very much how quickly the sow is dried off. Suddenly increasing the food when she is still milking may only stimulate the flow, which is undesirable. If she is on the point of drying off when the piglets are weaned, then she should receive an increasing ration within three to four days afterwards so that when she is served she will be getting from 6 to 7 lb (2·7 to 3 kg) of food.

Flushing gilts, however, is also important. It will pay you to give special attention to this point. Make it a practice to increase their food supply for a week or so before service. If a gilt due for service is a little low in condition, step up her ration by 1 or 2 lb (0·45 to 0·90 kg) of meal or nuts a little earlier than usual, but at all costs avoid getting her too fat.

High-level feeding should be continued for the first four weeks of pregnancy, reduced during the middle period and then increased during the last six weeks, rising to 8 lb (3·6 kg) per day for a large sow at the point of farrowing. The latter increase is to keep pace with the growth potential of the piglets which is remarkable during the last few weeks.

A more uniform system of feeding may be employed but the sow must be 25-30 lb (11-13·6 kg) heavier at each succeeding weaning. A properly compounded breeders' ration is essential, and for good measure some breeders give a multi-vitamin injection as soon as the in-pig animal is brought in to farrow. The quality of the colostrum will thereby be improved. Giving the same vitamin A, D and E mixture at weaning is said to improve fertility.

THE THIN SOW SYNDROME

A thin sow is no uncommon sight. At the end of lactation many sows are in low condition and if feeding has been inadequate they can look positively unthrifty. Some may be suffering from lung or kidney trouble and so fail to put on flesh. This sort of condition has long been recognised, but in the early 60s reports began to come in of sows going thin in batches after farrowing. There might be a dozen or even several score of sows affected at the same time. The trouble is worst in winter.

Sows, more often than gilts, rapidly lose flesh until they are virtually walking "toast-racks". The skin is dry and sometimes scaly, but appetite is maintained, milk production does not suffer if pigs are suckling, and the sows look generally alert. Many, however, do not come into season for some time after weaning, and many animals are grossly anaemic.

Because sow stalls were just coming into vogue at the time many people suggested that this system created a state of restlessness with consequent unthriftiness. But it is by no means always found associated with stalls. The problem seems to have arisen when there was a country-wide change of feeding regime, using a lower quantity than was traditional. But the quality was not adjusted accordingly, hence the development of what virtually was an under-feeding problem.

Most critical period for this breakdown is after weaning when body reserves are at their lowest. This is also the time when worm infestation is likely to reach a peak (see page 108).

Egg laying increases rapidly from shortly before farrowing and is maintained at a high level until lactation ceases. This, combined with the discovery of a worm burden in a great many very thin sows, makes one suspect that internal parasites play a part in creating this syndrome. They cause marked gastritis and a variable degree of damage to the mucous membrane of the bowel. A good response to the feeding of milk products, especially whey, and an injection of vitamin A supports the view that poor nutrition was to blame in the past.

General experience suggests that inadequate feeding is the basic cause of the trouble.

Stone-eating is often encountered and seems to be an attempt at compensation when appetite is unsatisfied and especially when parasites are present. In the latter circumstance anoestrus is a common feature.

Cold, rigorous surroundings are accepted as aggravating causes since they use up food for heat production rather than body building. The low levels of feeding often recommended will, in fact, reduce the thickness of backfat and so exaggerate heat loss.

Underfeeding during pregnancy can easily and automatically be compensated for by good feeding during lactation, but if during the latter period there is no opportunity for building up reserves, and putting on that 30 lb (13·6 kg) extra bodyweight at the end of each successive lactation, then a decline will set in which is very difficult in practice to put right. Recovery almost invariably is a slow process lasting about six months. Severely affected sows do not justify treatment and they should be culled, but for less advanced cases an improved feeding regime, with special reference to the energy value, should be accompanied by better housing. The important thing is never to let your sows get in low condition. An early diagnosis is also important.

At weaning a sow should not be in such a low "hat-rack" condition that she cannot recover quickly. Normally she will do so on a good sow ration, even if the food has to be cut down a little for three or four days to help stop the milk flow.

A gilt in high condition may first come into season at about six months of age.

But the prevalence of small gilt litters may well be due to too early service. So serve by weight rather than age and regard 200 lb (90 kg) as a minimum weight. If in good condition, serve at the second strong heat after this weight has been reached.

THE SEX CYCLE

Now just a few points about the service itself.

The sex cycle in a female pig is a regular process. Each complete cycle occupies from 15 to 30 days and averages about 21 days. It is broken up into the following phases:

Anoestrus (or quiescence)—8–10 days.

Proestrus (or preparation)—3 days.

Oestrus (the heat period)—3 days.

Metoestrus (returning to resting if no conception)—7 days.

During the three-day heat period, up to 25 follicles mature in the ovary. These rupture one after the other between the

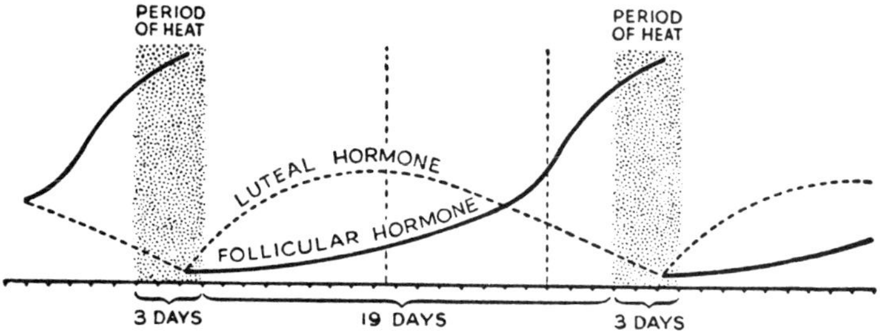

25th and 26th hour of the period and they travel down the Fallopian tubes towards the uterus.

During the latter part of their journey they meet with the sperm of the boar and become fertilised, finally settling in the womb and developing there.

The diagram shows how this sex (oestrous) cycle progresses.

You will note the point I have made about the shedding of eggs from the ovary between the 25th and 26th hour of the heat period.

Now suppose you have a sow or gilt served immediately she

comes into season. In such a case the boar's sperms have to wait in the female reproductive tract a considerable time before the eggs are available for fertilising.

Because of this there would be a risk that the virility of the sperms might decline and that some of the eggs would not be properly fertilised. In other words, the sow would have a smaller litter than she was capable of producing.

So a delay in service is advisable. But don't leave it too late.

To cover the full period of ova shedding and achieve maximum fertilation, it is best to allow first service at about 12-14 hours after the onset of heat and repeat 24 hours later (36 hours after onset).

The size of the litter born is, however, generally determined partly by genetical and partly by nutritional factors. It is known that a number of embryos die early in pregnancy, which (since they need little nutrition at this stage) seems to be due to some qualitative deficiency—perhaps an inadequate supply of some growth-stimulating substance—or to the distribution of the blood supply in the uterus. Rest and quiet for 2–3 weeks after service is now known to ensure maximum litter size by ensuring the establishment of the maximum number of ova on the womb bed.

Whilst heavy feeding may not directly influence the number of piglets born, it ensures that the pig can make use of its full potential. Heavier feeding in the later stages is likely, however, to ensure that more piglets are born alive and of good weight (3 lbs, 1·4 kg)—a very important survival factor.

RECOGNISING HEAT PERIOD

Recognition of the heat period is usually not difficult. The animal is sleepy and will lie about if on her own. With other pigs she may be noisy and restless, often mounting them and standing to be mounted. There is frequently a thick transparent mucous discharge from the vulva, sometimes bloodstained.

The ultimate test that a sow is ready for service is her willingness to allow an attendant to ride her; it is usually associated with a tensing and stiffening of her body when firm finger pressure is applied downwards in the loin region.

In a high percentage of female pigs a heat period occurs about three days after farrowing, three weeks later and in any case from 5 to 10 days after the piglets have been removed. Indications that this may be so may not be obvious and the phenomenon may pass unnoticed unless there is a boar close by. The sight and sound, and in particular contact with the boar tend to shorten the period from weaning to oestrus.

Mating in pigs is a prolonged process. It may continue for as long as 10 or 15 minutes after the boar has mounted the sow. About half-way through the boar relaxes and often appears to be very sleepy. This is a sign that matters are proceeding normally.

Don't interrupt the mating. The pair should be allowed to indulge in any preliminary love-making and they should be left entirely alone until they separate of their own free will.

The boar's ejaculate is large, being anything up to 500 ml in volume and consisting of different fractions. In general the appearance is of a milky fluid in which there is a large clot of gelatinous material. The sperms are unevenly distributed throughout the fluid portion, varying from 50 to 250 million per ml. The jelly-like clot occupies about one-third of the total volume.

On the farm some sows are very reluctant to take the boar even though penned in with him for several days. This, however, is infinitely better than just introducing the boar when the sow seems to be on heat. Leaving the two together generally results in several services, one of which is more likely to be at the optimal time than if the boar is brought in at an arbitrary time selected by the operator. Mating may be encouraged by spraying with an on-heat spray or introducing the smell, sight or grunt of the boar. Any sows that don't come on can be injected with a hormone and given an intramuscular injection of 100,000 units of vitamin A. Over-fat animals tend to be difficult to get into pig, whilst those in lean, hard condition cause no trouble.

If conception takes place, the sex cycle of the sow is broken

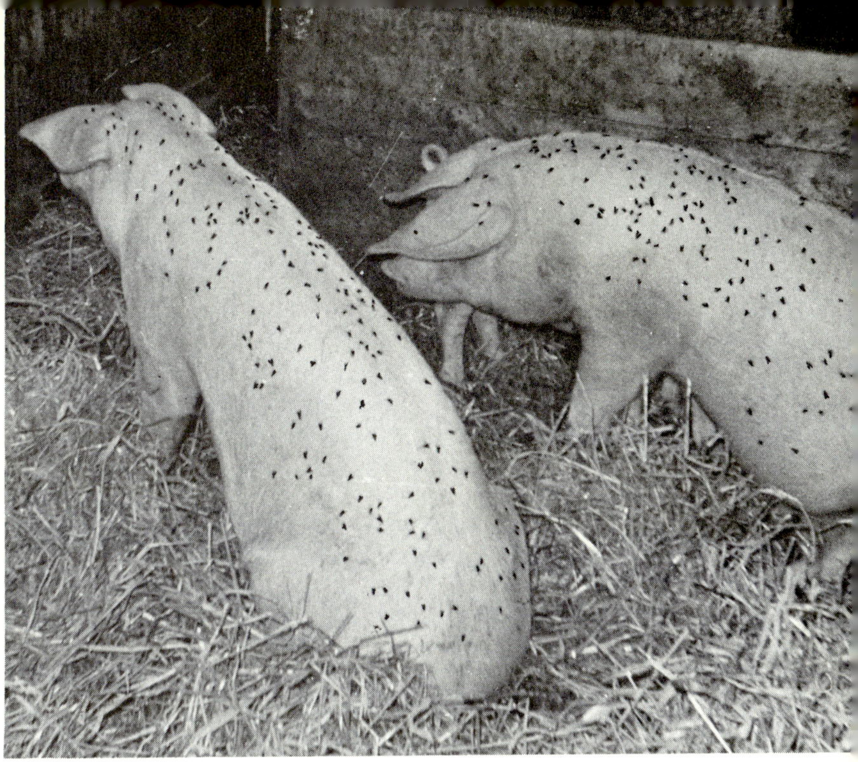

Flies in fattening pens can spread disease and should be controlled with a knock-down fly spray.

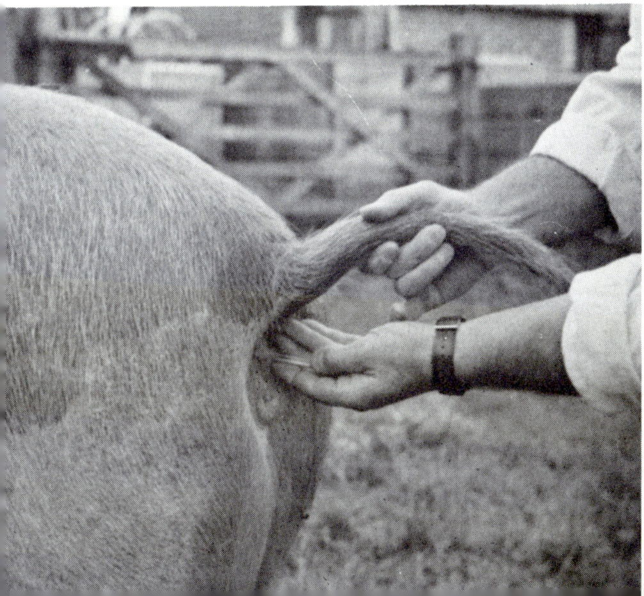

Temperature can be taken by inserting thermometer in pig's rectum.

Injecting a

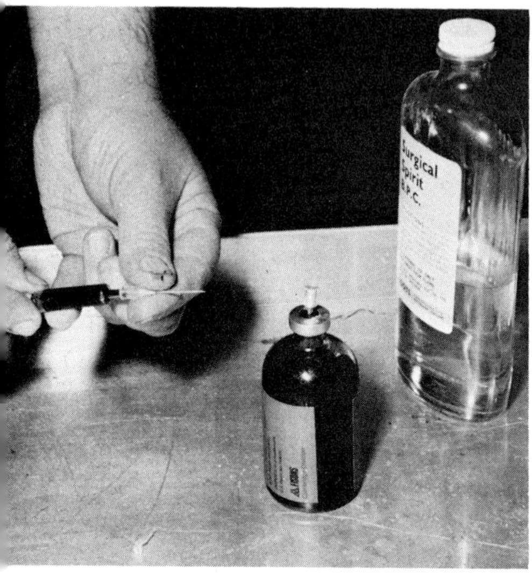

Use a disposable plastic hypodermic syringe with a 19-gauge (1.1 mm) bore, 12.5 mm (long) needle. Change needle after each litter.

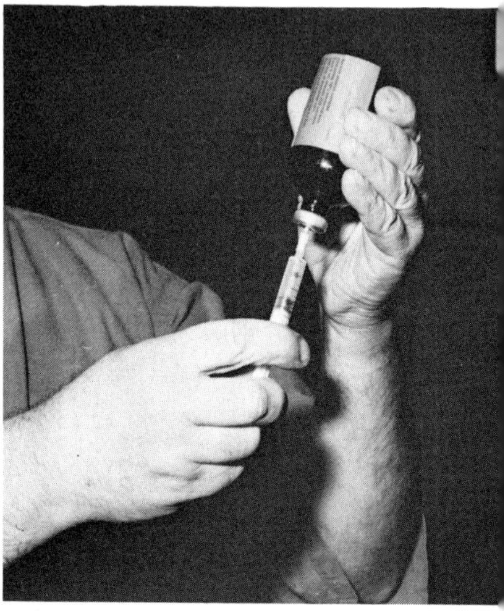

Fix syringe to needle already in bottle an inject 2 cc of air—to avoid creating vacuu when the iron solution is withdrawn.

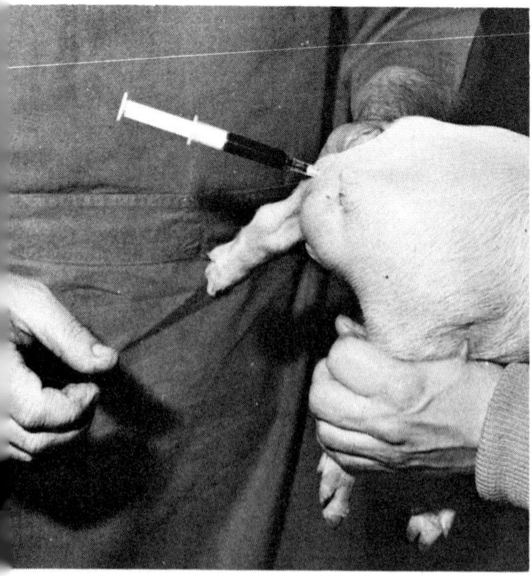

Tense skin over injection site and move it slightly sideways. Swab with surgical spirit and insert needle into ham.

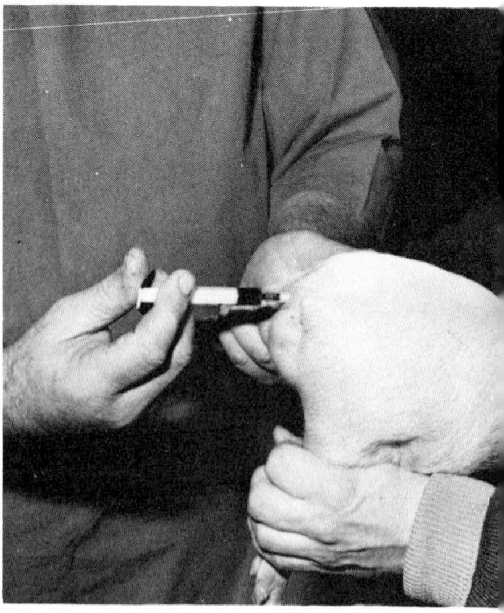

Depress plunger slowly to expel iron pre aration.

nst anaemia

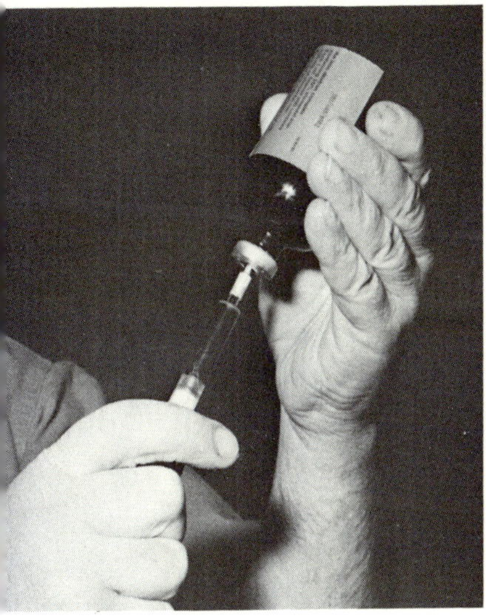

Hold bottle upside-down and draw out plunger slowly.

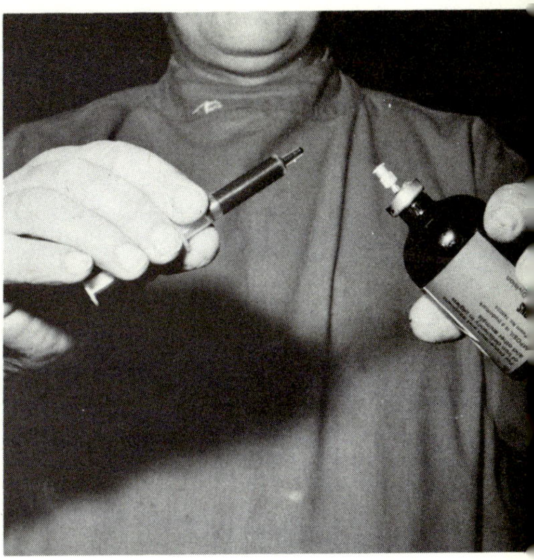

To avoid spillage lower the bottle before removing syringe.

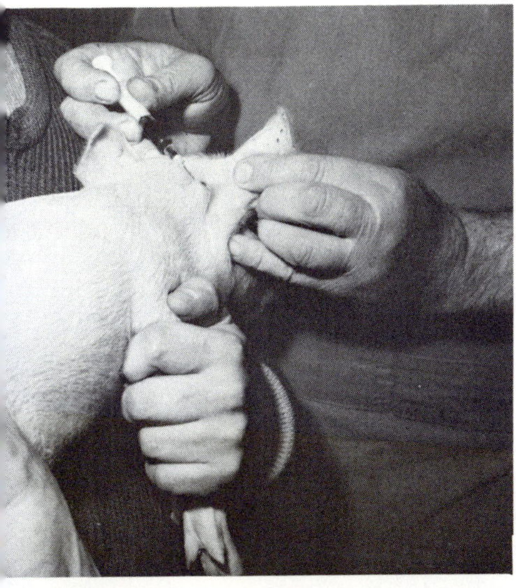

Subcutaneous iron injections are given just behind the ear. Insert needle almost parallel to skin to avoid going into pad of fat.

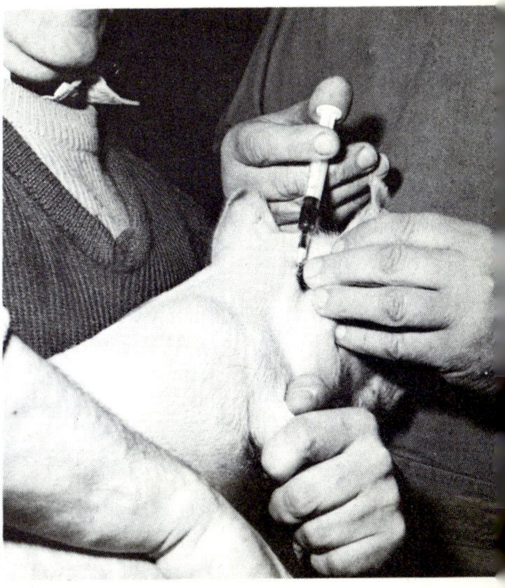

After needle is withdrawn, gently massage the area to disperse fluid.

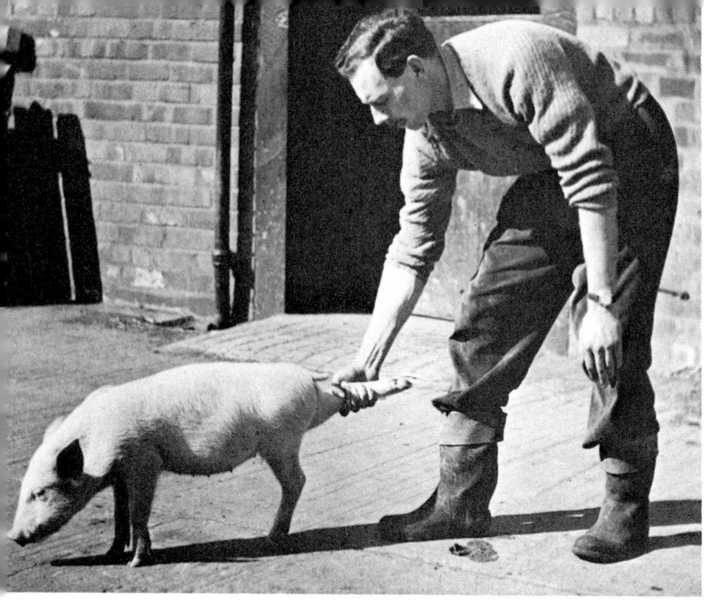

Correct way to catch and pick up a young pig.

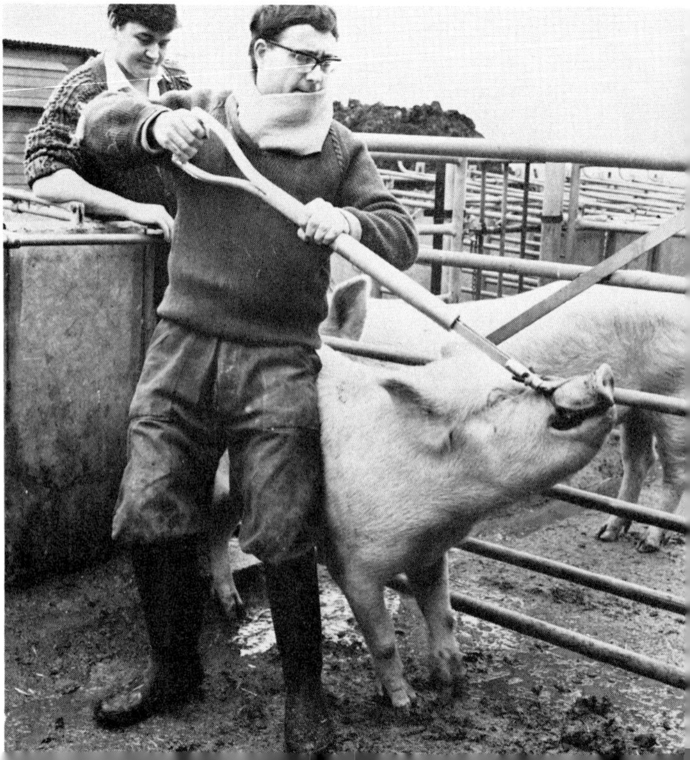

When length of stout wire is pulled through tubular handle of this pig holder it locks noose over pig's snout.

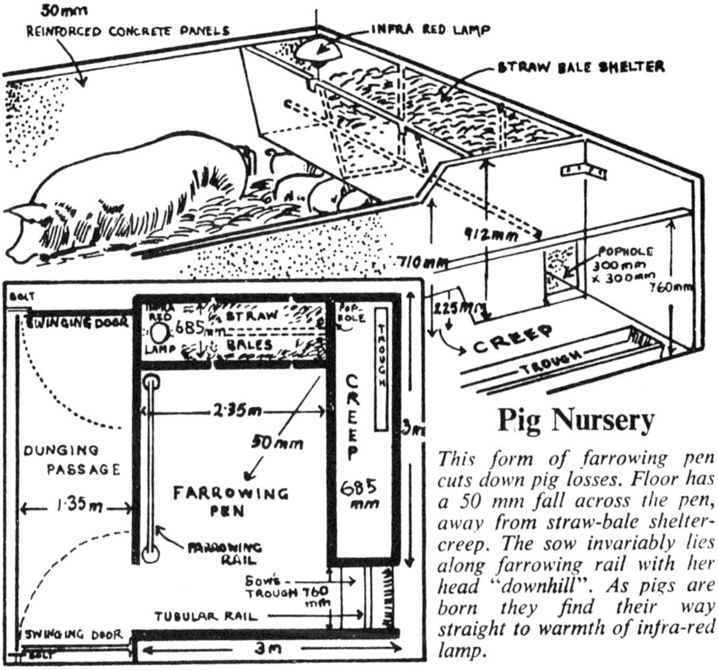

Pig Nursery

This form of farrowing pen cuts down pig losses. Floor has a 50 mm fall across the pen, away from straw-bale shelter-creep. The sow invariably lies along farrowing rail with her head "downhill". As pigs are born they find their way straight to warmth of infra-red lamp.

until after farrowing. She will not come in heat again until she has farrowed. But if the service is unsuccessful, the cycle will continue its usual course and "heat" will recur in about 21 days.

SERVING SOWS EARLIER

The development of satisfactory sowmilk substitutes and attractive creep foods which enable good litter weights to be achieved, irrespective of the sow's milk yield, has encouraged a great interest in systems of early weaning (see chapter 5) which enable a slightly increased turnover to take place by serving the sows earlier.

It must be remembered that the oestrus cycle is fundamentally a three-week cycle, with the sow tending to come into season every three weeks from the third day after farrowing. Therefore, from a practical point of view, it is desirable to wean about a week before anticipated oestrus to get the best results.

AVOIDING CONCEPTION DELAYS

Five-week weaning is thus more satisfactory than four-week weaning, because it enables the sow to adjust herself, lose her milk, and come in at six weeks. Adherence to this physiological fact will reduce the risks of "turning", and avoid delays in conception.

Many sows and gilts actually come into physiological heat at the times mentioned, though this may not be evident unless a boar is near at hand. He will then show signs of interest and the sow will become agitated.

Service at three weeks three days can be successful. If the sows are removed from their litters no change in the feeding regime is needed, but, if, as is not uncommon, the boar is let in with a bunch of sows and their litters, a few more pounds (kg) of food for each sow per day for several days before anticipated heat (or up to day of service), seems to be important.

TESTS FOR PREGNANCY

To ascertain whether the sow has held to service or not, an injection of one milligramme of stilboestrol may be given 16 days after. This is best carried out after the first heat period has passed. If she comes into season in a few days, then she should be served again as this shows that she has not held. If, however, there is no reaction, she can be presumed to be in pig.

If X-ray equipment is available, then evidence of pregnancy can be secured after one week. A very effective method, though one which requires laboratory facilities and a knowledge of histology, involves snipping a minute portion of tissues from the forward part of the vaginal cervix, using an instrument with a sliding rod cutting edge. This is effective 30-50 days after service.

Tissue from the cervix in the empty animal is characterised by 20 or more uneven layers of irregularly-placed, variable-shaped large cells covering the lining surface, whereas in the pregnant animal it has only two or three layers of regularly-distributed prominent cells.

There is also the highly practical method of manual manipulation via the rectum. In the pregnant animal as might be expected the uterine artery is prominent and can be easily compared after some experience has been gained, with the external iliac artery on the same side. The former develops a vibration or 'fremitus'.

Finally, the ultrasonic method of detecting foetal pulse can be employed with success and can be tried from 4–5 weeks after service.

All these methods of course are clearly ones for the expert to apply but their intelligent use can undoubtedly save time, embarrassment and money. But you should consider the benefit of adopting pregnancy diagnosis as a routine.

INFERTILITY

In the pig infertility is becoming an increasingly serious problem. Sometimes gilts may fail to come into season because the weather is too cold, or they may be held in dark sheds for long periods. By bringing them indoors and putting them under a bright lamp for a week heat may be induced. The light factor here may be as important as in other animals. Walk the boar past the pen twice daily and notice how the gilts react.

The sound, smell and contact with a boar stimulates sexual interest and encourages ovulation. The salival froth of the boar contains the hormone androstinal which further encourages oestrus.

If you have more than one returning, do not overlook the fact that the boar may be responsible; so rest him for several weeks or, if you suspect he is defective have his semen examined. Sometimes a young boar may show lack of interest due to extreme youth; more often this is the aftermath of previous mismanagement. Faulty feeding, bad feet, a fall due to a slippery floor, or an attack by a sow not properly in heat, can all make the youngster shy of his work. Incompatibility in the relative size and shape of the genital organs may result in repeated faulty service, ejaculation taking place into the rectum. So observe service very carefully.

It may be that a number of females fail to show heat or to hold to service all at one time. They could be over-fat, a circumstance which invariably appears to be associated with poor conception. On the other hand they may be suffering from the thin sow syndrome (see page 44). Removing anoestrus animals from one pen to another creates stress, which often precipitates oestrus.

FAILURE TO CONCEIVE

Failure to conceive may also be associated with the presence of an intercurrent disease such as an attack of erysipelas. Fortunately the venereal diseases encountered in cattle such as trichomoniasis and vibrio foetus infection of the womb do not occur in the pig, though it is possible at times an infection of the womb with a virus or a mycoplasma may cause disturbance.

An intramuscular injection of vitamin A* appears to have an overall beneficial effect where heat periods are absent or irregular and for which there is no obvious explanation. When parasites are present this procedure is still worthwhile since in these circumstances vitamin A is rapidly leached out of the liver and the inflammation caused by the parasites tends to interfere with assimilation. (See also SMEDI virus, page 60.)

SYRINGING

Where there is some cloudy discharge syringing the passage out with a mild disinfectant solution such as Dettol (20 ml to half a litre of water) is useful. This should be followed by inserting an antiseptic cone as far as possible into the passage with the fingers. Repeat this treatment every three or four days until the discharge clears. In these circumstances, a course of penicillin injections over three or four days, coupled with a 10-grain tablet of potassium iodide per day for a similar period will help.

In more stubborn cases of sterility, veterinary advice is best sought for valuable animals; others are best got into good condition and slaughtered.

* *100,000 units.*

USING A BOAR

A young boar of eight months of age should start with not more than three gilts a week, later being given four. Use him first on an old sow as first services generally produce small litters. When mature, one boar should be allowed for every 20 females.

If he is reluctant to serve, examine him carefully for painful joints, swollen sheath, etc, and if he shows a lack of sexual interest, check on his feeding and give him extra vitamin A or an injection of 100,000 units of this vitamin. Deficiency of vitamin A may also lead to sterility. If necessary, arrange for your veterinary surgeon to have him injected with a suitable hormone.

If in doubt about the efficiency of the boar, try another boar to determine where the fault lies.

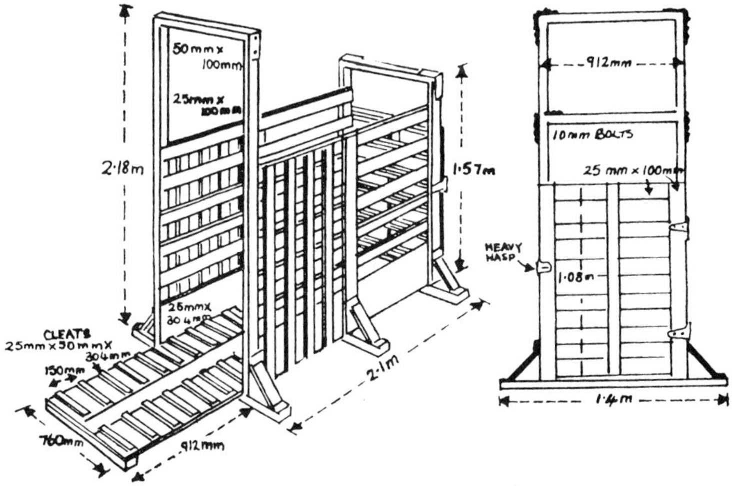

USEFUL SERVICE CRATE

The boar is supported on two 50 mm x 1·8 m planks, the front ends of which rest on gate and the rear ends on cleated floor. Adjust height of the front ends to suit the boar; then insert 50 x 100 mm bar through crate sides and under planks. (N.B. Planks are removable and are not shown in this constructional drawing.)

Poor breeding records can be as much a result of bad management as of poor animals. Proper feeding and housing are important for both sexes.

ARTIFICIAL INSEMINATION

Over the past few years considerable attention has been paid to the economic advantages of employing the technique of artificial insemination in pigs. Whilst much has been learnt from the allied field of cattle insemination, the problems of the pig are different and pose considerable difficulties.

In the first instance it is not so easy to persuade the boar to serve, but a padded wooden artificial structure scented with sow urine is now in wide use and with the apparatus employed enables the collection of voluminous semen which the boar produces at each ejaculation. Optimum semen collection intervals appear to be between five and six days, although this can be done at three-day intervals with some boars. Nevertheless, increasing frequency of collection may result in a rise in the percentage of abnormal spermatozoa. The ejaculate which may reach 500 c.c. in volume comprises various fractions, varying from a thin translucent fluid to much thicker portions containing great concentrations of sperm, together with a "granular" gelatinous fraction somewhat resembling frog's spawn, which is liberated continuously through the process of ejaculation. The latter seems to prevent the backward flow of the semen from the cervical region, which has no restrictive collar such as is found in the cow. When the animal is fully in season the lumen of the cervical tube somewhat resembles a corkscrew and so locks firmly with the penis when this is inserted. This no doubt is also a mechanism for preventing the backwards discharge of semen.

The semen itself is by no means as robust as that of the bull, and though there has been improvement in techniques of storage and diluents—such as yolk citrate glucose, and skim milk and glycerine, much has yet to be learnt about conservation. But it is now possible to preserve semen by freezing so that it can be sent through the post.

Some 60 to 100 ml. is a satisfactory volume for insemination with good quality diluted semen, but the problem is to ascertain the exact period when the sow is fully in season. It is said that ovulation occurs from 25 to 26 hours after the onset of heat and the survival of the ova is from 10 to 21 hours. It must be borne in mind that the spermatozoa take some time to reach the Fallopian tube. This is estimated to be about 13 hours, although they may survive for nearly four times as long. However, their fertilising capacity is retained for only 24 to 32 hours; the optimum insemination time therefore is considered to be from 10 to 26 hours after the onset of heat. The collection of semen, storage and insemination constitute a precise operation.

CONCEPTION PROSPECTS

One of the practical difficulties to be faced is the accurate assessment of the heat period and this, with the obvious difficulties of standardising the whole procedure, makes the fluctuations in conception rate understandable. A good rate would be over 70 per cent to first insemination, and poor ones, which are not uncommon, would be as low as 40 per cent. A really successful rate can only be achieved by eliminating those animals whose state of ovulation appears to be in doubt. When every animal on the farm is served on chance, then the conception rate is likely to be low.

Pigs fully on heat stand firmly on all four legs, allow themselves to be ridden, and dip their backs when finger pressure is applied over the loins. Insemination at this stage gives optimum results, although the percentage success is markedly reduced if pigs move during the insemination. The reaction to pressure applied to the back is most marked 24 to 36 hours after the onset of heat. Increasing success in the presence or proximity of a boar suggests that sound and smell encourage the pressure response.

As a process for improving a blood line, and avoiding the introduction of disease by bringing fresh animals on to the place, artificial insemination has much to recommend it. The transport of semen, and the whole technique of insemination, have, however, reached a high standard of proficiency.

PREPARING SOW FOR FARROWING

Only in rare cases, and perhaps more often in gilts, is it necessary to bring animals in to farrow sooner than a week before farrowing is due. The less time they are left to spend inside the better, for they tend to become lethargic and disinclined to take exercise and therefore less food and water. Sows today acclimatise themselves very quickly to their farrowing quarters.

The importance of proper housing has already been stressed in chapter 2. But again I emphasise how much a satisfactory farrowing house will help you in avoiding losses.

Before the sow moves in, it is well to clean out the house thoroughly. If the pen is caked with dung and dust, soak the walls and floor, scrape them and then scrub them with scalding soda water (one handful of washing soda to 1 gall (4·5 litres) of boiling water). This reduces the concentration of *E. coli.*

At this stage—*i.e.* one week before farrowing—the sow can be wormed. She can be given a dose of a remedy in her food that will affect all the parasites involved. It is not necessary to starve the animal beforehand.

Twenty-four hours later the pig should be thoroughly cleansed. Her underparts and backside should be washed with soap and water to remove dung. In this way worm eggs (discussed fully in chapter 7) are also removed, and the baby pigs are protected from infestation.

If lice parasites are present, the sow's back should be smeared liberally with pig oil. Let it cover a good three inches (75 mm) either side of the backbone from behind the neck to the tail. Alternatively, a mange dressing can be sprayed on. The ears should be swabbed out as this is the common reservoir of these parasites.

All this should, of course, be done before the sow is moved to clean farrowing quarters.

Try and avoid any violent change in the animal's diet. If she came in from grass, see that she has some cut grass or other green food every day. Lucerne is particularly good in this respect; kale is excellent in winter.

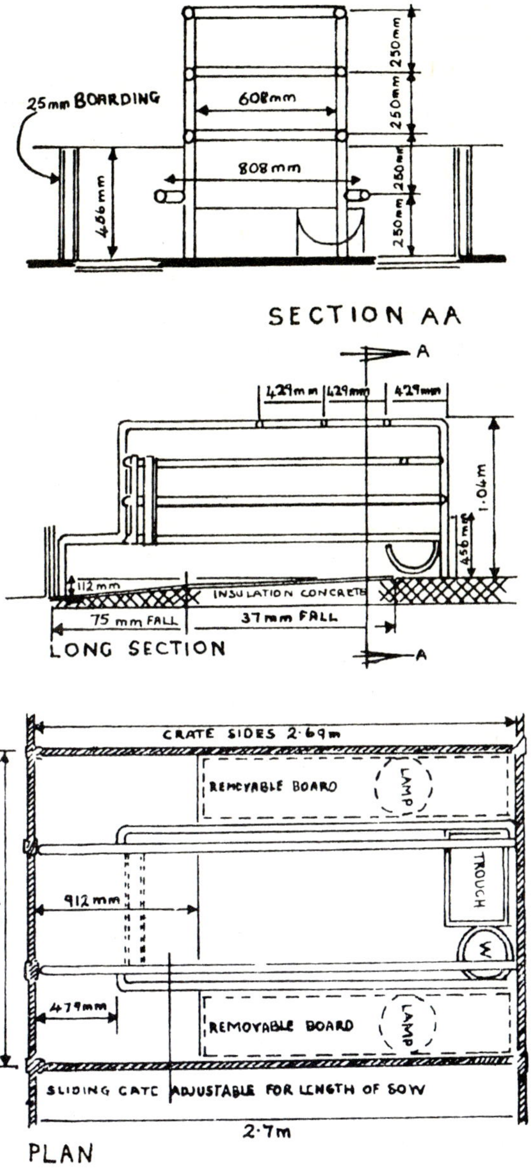

A tubular farrowing stall designed by the Farm Buildings Department, North of Scotland College of Agriculture.

FEEDING ROUTINE

Fresh green foods in small quantities at this stage serve to maintain interest and appetite apart from having somewhat laxative qualities. The following feeding routine is, however, to be recommended at this stage. From the day the sow is put into the farrowing pen, cut down the food by 1 lb ($\frac{1}{2}$ kg) a day to as little as $2\frac{1}{4}$ lb (1 kg). At this stage, to satisfy appetite, it may be necessary to double up with bran. Mix half this with $2\frac{1}{2}$-$3\frac{1}{2}$ galls (10-15 litres) of water night and morning. This method will ensure that adequate water is taken, which is so essential from the milk production point of view. In winter the water should have the chill taken off it.

The bowels can be kept open by 2 oz (60 ml) of pig oil each day or a $\frac{1}{4}$ lb (113 g) of Epsom salts on one day, although the bran will itself open the ration and help to keep the dung loose.

Another matter that needs attention before farrowing is the bedding. If the farrowing house is not heated, then straw could be used as bedding. So long as her movements are restricted, piglets appear to be perfectly able to find their way about, even in long straw, and avoid being laid on. Chaff and shavings or sawdust make good litter, and reduce knee and pastern blisters caused when piglets are struggling for a teat. The creep area should be warm and litter here is unnecessary.

FARROWING

Indication of impending farrowing is an increased swelling and flabbiness of the vulva. Milk appears in the teats about 12 hours before farrowing; about six hours before the event the sow may get down into a recumbent position and, from this stage onwards, will usually refuse food.

From the onset of labour you can usually, but by no means always, reckon the job will be over in about two hours. It may be all over in an hour or it may occasionally last for 12 or more. It pays to have someone in attendance at farrowings. That extra piglet can often be saved.

For example, piglets usually come without their envelopes; but, should any be delivered still encased, these envelopes must be removed—otherwise suffocation will result. Usually the cord does not need much attention, but if in doubt, dry it off with sulphonamide powder.

Without artificial warmth in cold weather, the piglets will naturally seek the warmth of the sow's body. Then they may be inadvertently killed through overlying. So take all the steps you can to guard against these losses.

Whilst in winter a lamp may be needed until the piglets are several weeks of age, in summer conditions may allow it to be turned off after a few days. It is essential that the creep nest is box-like and well-lit. Bars alone, across a corner, will *not* do. Cold air is drawn across the floor and the corner made colder. Don't have the lamps too low or the piglets may be scorched. Usually 12″-18″ (300 mm-460 mm) above the animals is about right, but check by hand after the lamps have been on for 10-15 minutes.

PIGLETS BORN DEAD

Where the sow is ill, especially when she has a high temperature, as in cases of swine fever and erysipelas, abortion may occur. This is, however, a rare occurrence although it may result from bad handling or recent transportation. There is no infectious abortion recognised in this country comparable to contagious abortion in cows. Piglets may, however, be slipped as a result of a vitamin A deficiency. Where leptospira infection occurs in the second half of pregnancy abortion may occur (see leptospirosis in chapter 7).

If the piglets inside the womb are dead, the sow loses her appetite and appears off colour. An injection of penicillin and one of stilboestrol may be tried in this case. Whilst the cause should be investigated, it is not usual for an animal to repeat this performance at her next farrowing.

Dead full-term piglets may be associated with prolonged farrowing, very large litters of over 17 or 18, a low protein intake during the last month of pregnancy, a vitamin A deficiency or a disturbance in iodine metabolism. In pigs kept intensively an iodine or an iron deficiency may arise if there is insufficient in the diet. A high calcium intake may have a similar effect and can be aggravated by providing chalk lumps on the pastures or the feeding of excessive quantities of a mineral mixture.

THE SMEDI VIRUS

Losses at farrowing time are much on the increase due to the spread of a virus known as the SMEDI virus. The letters stand for "stillbirths, mummies and repeated turnings to service".

Clearly this is a very unpleasant infection to have. Piglets may arrive dark brown in colour, shrivelled up or just dead and looking normal. Litters may arrive early or late and only a small number of individuals may be mummies.

The sows appear unaffected but the effects of the virus are far-reaching. There will be false pregnancies, increased returns to service, small litters with the above abnormalities, and some of those born alive will be weak, often displaying splay leg and trembles.

After an attack immunity develops in a herd in a matter of months. But every effort should nevertheless be made to limit the spread, by batch farrowing. Unfortunately there are at least four types of entero-viruses, so several similar attacks can be experienced and infection can be spread by AI.

It must be noted here that similar misfortunes may follow an outbreak of TGE, where the sows have become affected but show little or no symptoms themselves.

HOLDING PIGLETS

If you do attend a farrowing and have cause to handle the pigs, take care how you pick them up, not necessarily for the pig's sake, but for your own! A squeaking piglet may easily upset the sow and that may completely disorganise the farrowing. It may cause cannibalism; it could, at the worst, lead to the sow attacking you.

So grasp the piglet by the snout, keeping its mouth shut so that it cannot squeal; at the same time put your other hand beneath its belly to lift it.

There is no need to dry the youngsters. They will dry off

remarkably quickly if left alone, especially where there is the attraction of a heated corner; they will go to it and will then come out and suck when they feel like it.

FARROWING COMPLICATIONS

Sometimes a farrowing is protracted. One or two pigs may be dropped and a delay of up to several hours may occur before the rest are delivered.

You can easily tell if there are more to come; the sow will be unlikely to get up and will take no notice of the piglets already born. But, as a general rule, you should be suspicious of trouble if she goes more than six hours without making an effort to produce the rest of the piglets.

You should also suspect trouble if the sow strains for more than half-an-hour without effect. The most likely trouble would be two piglets coming together and forming an obstruction in the passage. In such a case help would be necessary.

If you have any doubts about tackling the job, call professional help without delay. But if you wish to try carefully yourself, thoroughly cleanse and soap your hand and arm and gently work your hand into the passage to try and release the obstruction. Usually farrowing will proceed normally after this action.

Should you get a complicated case where this sort of thing happens more than once, I strongly advise you to consider sending the sow for slaughter as soon as possible after farrowing Too much manual interference is quite likely to set up inflammation of the womb and lead sooner or later to a dead sow.

IN WINTER

Where no artificial heat is available for new-born piglets in winter—and especially when farrowing is protracted—it will pay to remove all bits of membrane and pieces of afterbirth from the youngsters, to dry them with a clean towel and place them in a cloth-lined basket with a covered hot-water bottle or a wrapped-up warm brick in the middle.

Should a weakly pig fail to start breathing, artificial respiration can be applied. Hold the animal with its head slightly downward, grip the chest firmly between thumb and fingers and apply gentle but firm pressure intermittently at the rate of about one squeeze every second. Or remove mucus from the mouth and apply the 'kiss of life'.

An afterbirth usually comes from a sow shortly after the last pig is born. It should be removed from the pen and buried or burnt so that the sow does not eat it.

Now all the actions I have suggested seem to indicate that farrowing is a complicated business and that constant attention is necessary. Actually it is only occasionally that intervention is essential. Even then it should be given with the minimum of fuss and disturbance to the sow, otherwise the quietest of sows may be upset.

So, as far as possible, keep in the background and only take action when things would go wrong if you did not give some help.

Most farmers like to use farrowing crates as a means of restraining a sow or gilt and making it more convenient to give a hand when occasion arises. It certainly reduces the risk of injury to piglets—especially when the sow it not a particularly good mother. They need not be complicated and many of the simpler ones are very effective, comfortable, safe and labour-saving.

Chapter 5

AFTER-FARROWING TROUBLES

We have dealt with the problems likely to arise up to and during farrowing. Now we come to the after-farrowing difficulties.

The first one you may meet is lack of milk in the sow. So, if you attend the farrowing, as soon as it is all over check up on the milk supply.

Normally you will find matters satisfactory. But if you can't draw any milk or can only get a little, gently massage the udder. This will often get things going and ensure a proper flow.

At this stage you can see many of the teats are actually giving milk. If there are fewer than the number of piglets in the litter, the surplus pigs should be removed and either given to another sow or reared artificially. The problem of artificial rearing is dealt with later in this chapter (see also blind teats under hereditary factors).

WHEN MILK FAILS

Sometimes there is no milk at all—a condition we do not yet understand properly. It is often associated with a series of events resembling milk fever in the cow. But we do know that in such cases a milk fever injection—about 250 c.c. of calcium borogluconate under the skin behind the ear—will help matters, particularly if an intravenous injection of pituitrin is given at the same time. This, of course, is a job for a veterinary surgeon.

But after the milk flow has started you can promote it (and the sow's appetite) by giving a warm bran mash containing a stimulant. Mix about 3 lb (1·36 kg) of bran with scalding water. Stir until cool enough for the sow to drink, then add $\frac{1}{4}$ oz (7 ml) of ammonium acetate solution. Vigorous massage is also useful.

This milk fever type of disease is often associated with the condition of the sow. It is more common in animals that have had insufficient exercise during the dry period, especially those that have been overfed and are over-fat. Lack of water, especially in winter time, is important.

Lack of Milk (Agalactia)

There are unfortunately many occasions when a sow or gilt reaches farrowing time and is unable to produce any milk. The litter may arrive and starve because there is no milk available in the udder, which appears otherwise normal. While the causes of such a deficiency are still not clear, observations show that certain circumstances predispose to this condition.

In over-fat sows a condition resembling acetonaemia has been recorded. This may occur just before or just after farrowing. Whilst the temperature is of no significance, there may be a considerable drowsiness, in some cases almost reaching a state of coma. The condition is most common where pigs have been heavily-fed with protein-rich feedingstuffs plus bulky foods such as potatoes, right up to the point of farrowing.

Sodium propionate treatment, at one-third the cattle dose, has been shown to be effective, as well as an increased vitamin D level in the food. Diagnosis and treatment should, however, be left in the hands of the veterinary surgeon.

On the other hand an unbalanced ration containing too much fibre, low in protein and lacking minerals and vitamins is known to encourage milk failure. Such a ration may occur under conditions of swill feeding when insufficient "balancer" meal is being provided. Swill is generally low in protein and minerals and is unlikely to contain either vitamin D or A. Care should

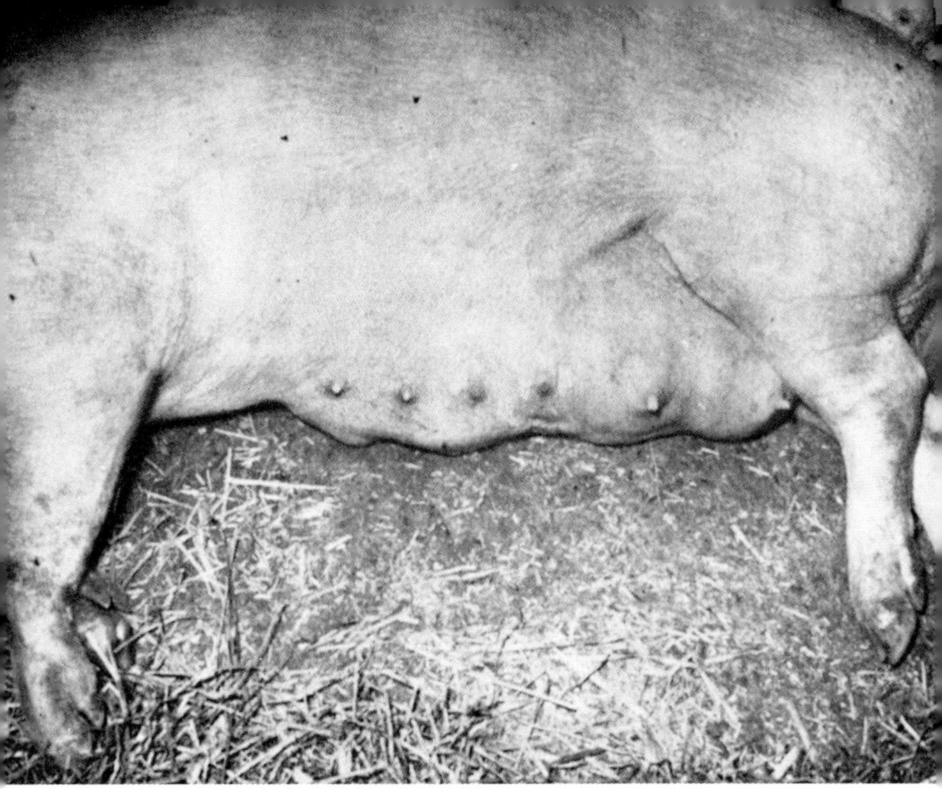

Sow suffering from mastitis—note hard, swollen quarters of her udder.

Farrowing fever makes this sow reluctant to rise and her pigs are unable to suckle.

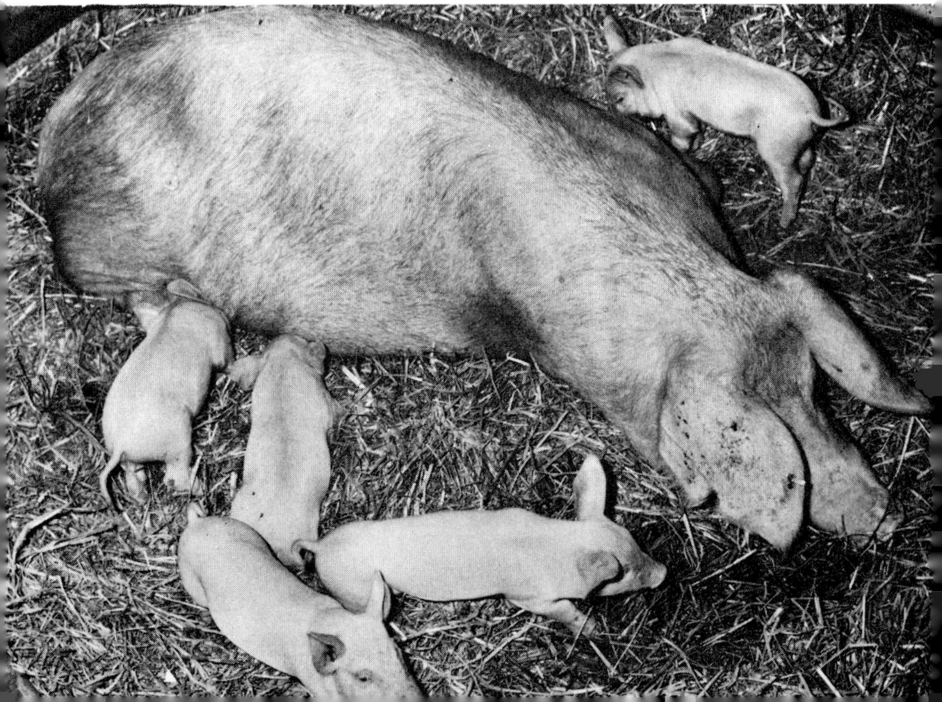

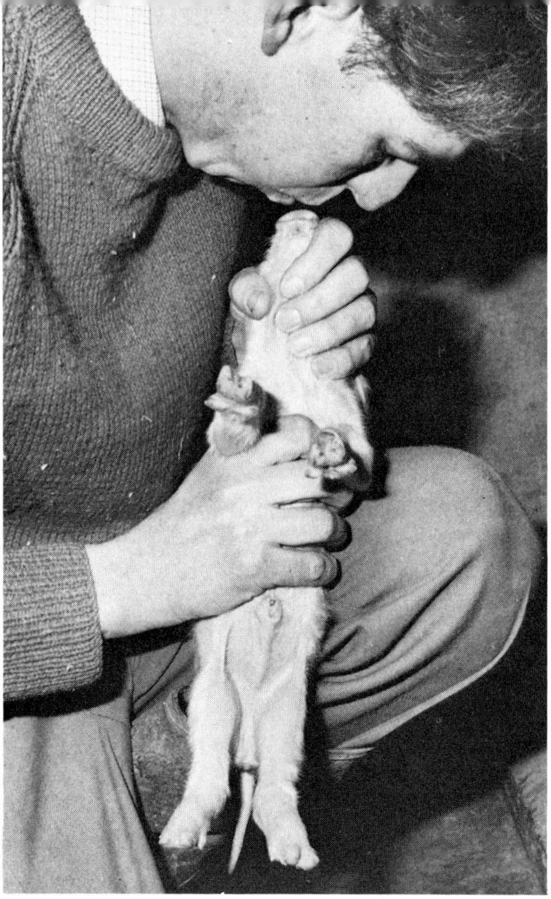

The 'kiss of life' will often revive a piglet that has been overlain by the sow.

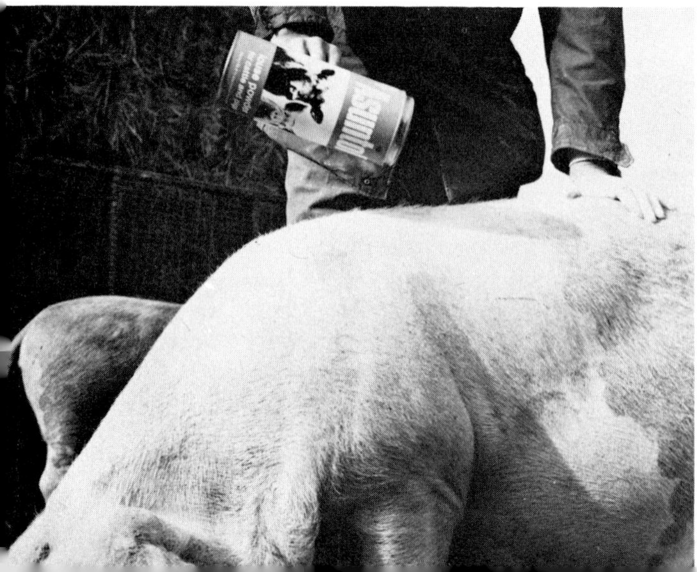

Breeding stock should be dressed routinely with lice powder.

Photo: Baywood Chemicals

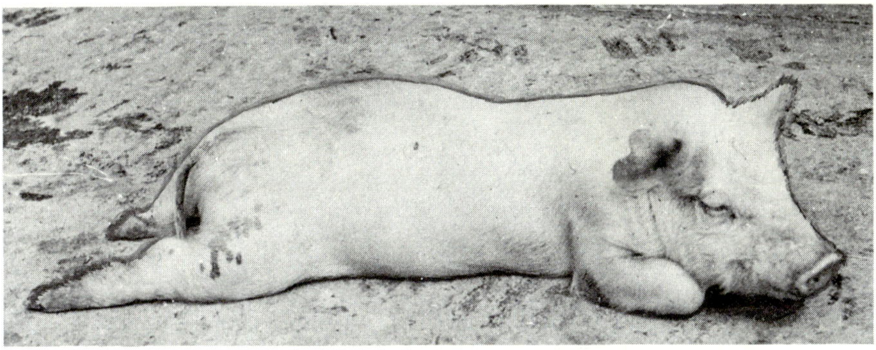

Posterior paralysis (above) of 3-week-old pig caused by vitamin A deficiency.

Piglet born without eyeballs (right) from sow deficient in vitamin A.

Photos by Dr R. F. Goodwin

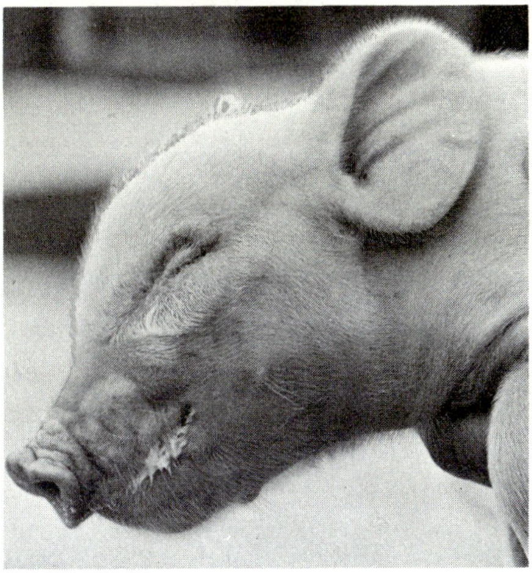

Typical 'goose-stepping' gait in baconer suffering from pantothenic acid deficiency.

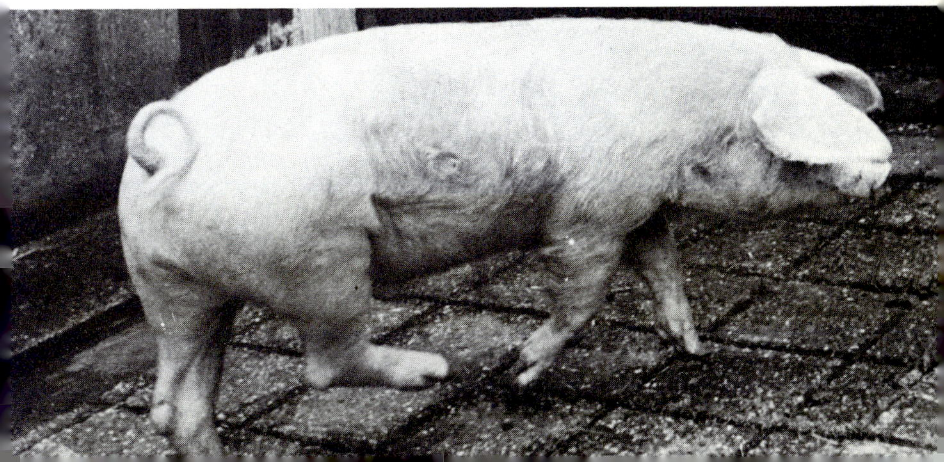

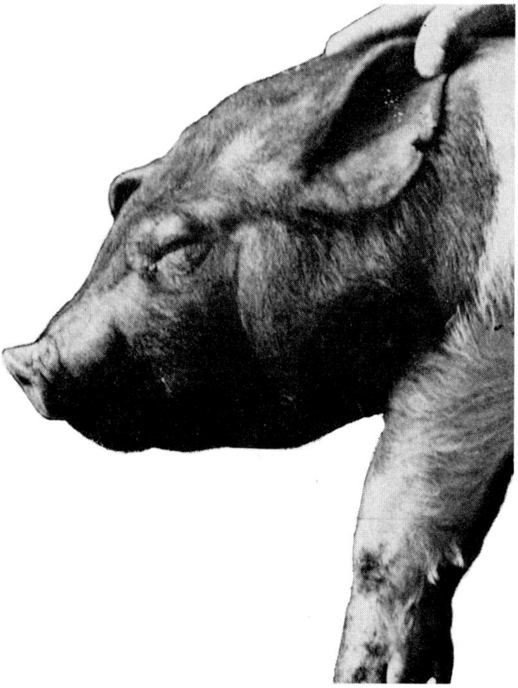

Puffiness around the eyes and snout is characteristic of bowel oedema.

Pigs suffering from necrotic enteritis, and sharing emaciated condition and stunted growth.

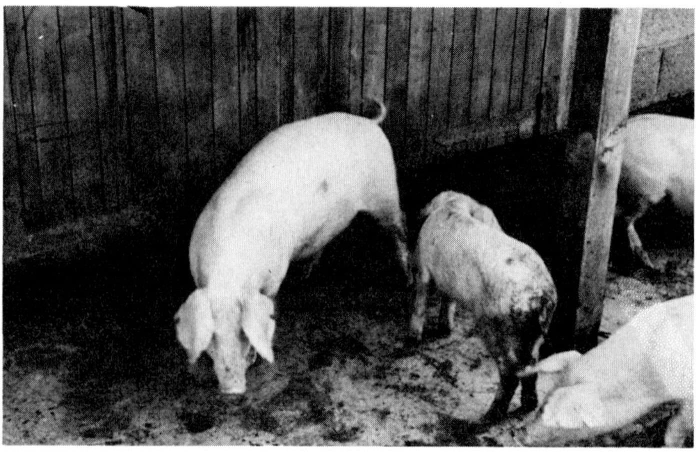

be taken, therefore, to balance up the swill with the necessary constituents, otherwise it is likely to cause an over-fat condition which is often associated with a poor milk yield. On the other hand, certain strains of pigs tend to be over-fat and to suffer more than others from agalactia.

Sometimes the trouble may be caused by lack of exercise and, in particular, insufficient water. But the provision of water bowls is not always a sure preventative, for they may not be used or may freeze up during cold weather.

If a sow is exposed to severe conditions and poorly fed, energy will be used up to keep the animal warm and the milk flow will suffer. This will likewise be adversely affected when disease is present. Contagious diseases, such as erysipelas or swine fever, are examples. Infection of the uterus after farrowing, mastitis and milk fever (to which we have already referred) are conditions associated with a lack of milk or complete milk failure.

Farrowing Fever

This omnibus heading covers a number of conditions or perhaps different aspects of one. Symptoms of milk fever or acetonaemia may exist; there is little or no milk and it is generally evident some days before the sow is due to farrow that she is suffering from discomfort. Her bag is firm, hard and hot. The condition is often associated with a whitish discharge from the vulva. Some authorities suspect that there is a sub-chronic endometritis or inflammation of the womb leading to a low-grade septicaemia. The sow is reluctant to rise, and if she does get up shows crampiness or discomfort as though suffering from laminitis—also known as fever of the feet. Her temperature may be slightly or markedly raised, varying from 103° to 106°F (40° to 41°C).

This condition is commonest where farrowing takes place indoors and is relatively rare where the breeding stock run out-of-doors and farrowing takes place in movable huts.

Whilst a true explanation of all cases is not possible, an organism known as klebsiella, closely related to *E. coli*, has been discovered in association with the damaged udder tissue in many cases and is considered to play a major part in this complex affliction. It thrives in the bowel and can be transmitted by contact and distributed in the dung. It should therefore be regarded as an infectious condition and treated accordingly.

Some cases may be due to a true coliform toxaemia. But whatever the cause, when the temperature is high, an injection of terramycin is usually effective.

The risk of this ailment can be reduced by keeping the sow (gilts are seldom affected) in good lean condition and preventing her from becoming lethargic by adopting the feeding and management regime prior to farrowing recommended in chapter 4.

Lack of water and a tendency to constipation appear to be two of the important factors which encourage this condition.

A few cases of agalactia due to ergot-contaminated feed have been recorded in this country. This particular plant fungus is widely distributed on our own grasses, such as ryegrass and Yorkshire fog, in early autumn, and may sometimes contaminate grain. Imported feedingstuffs may also be contaminated.

Mastitis (bacterial other than Klebsiella)

Yet another complication that may arise about this time is mastitis. This should be suspected when the quarters are irregularly swollen and when hard lumps can be felt deep in the tissue. Milk can only be drawn with difficulty from affected quarters. It usually contains clots or is watery and blood-stained.

Damage to the udder may be caused by the piglets' sharp teeth, so opening the way to mastitis-producing bacteria. Chaps and cracks may similarly be the starting point of infection. The latter can be treated by using a penicillin cream, or injecting an antibiotic deeply into the affected quarter. Sores may be produced by the udder rubbing on cold, damp concrete floors where there is insufficient bedding. The type of germ present is usually a staphylococcus, but this can be confirmed by sending a carefully taken sample of milk to a laboratory.

To prevent infection persisting in a latent form in the udder, an injection of penicillin directly into the tissues during the dry period may help.

As a rule piglets do not seem to suffer any immediate harm if they suckle affected quarters but, where practicable, it is advisable, for the sake of the sow, to keep them away for 24 hours whilst the quarters are being treated. Recovery is the usual experience.

Eversion or Prolapse of the Uterus

This is fairly common in sows either shortly before or immediately after farrowing. Over-fat sows, generally associated with faulty feeding, are the usual victims. A sudden fright during farrowing, causing this to be prolonged with consequent straining, may also precipitate this misfortune. It might also be caused by too heavy feeding with bulk foods prior to farrowing. To be effective, surgical interference must be applied by a veterinary surgeon within a few hours of the occurrence; the womb is generally turned inside out. When attended to early, it is possible to replace the organ satisfactorily. The operation can be done successfully under anaesthesia or with the use of the tranquilliser azaperone. But sometimes serious damage is done. Slaughter is then the best policy.

Cannibalism

A problem that can arise immediately after (or during) farrowing is cannibalism. This may not be due to any inherent vice in the sow. She may go to move a pig and, when lifting it in her mouth, taste blood. That may lead her to eat the pig and all the rest of the litter too.

While a well-designed farrowing pen will help to reduce the tendency for this habit to develop, the use of the farrowing crate or a pen with farrowing rails, as already indicated, will keep losses to a minimum. If a warm, illuminated creep is provided, piglets will tend to keep away from the sow except during actual suckling. Irritation caused by the sharp, uncut milk teeth may be another means of stimulating anger and induce snapping and savaging.

If you are present when the trouble starts, you must act quickly. The sow must be restrained and the piglets removed to allow the sow to relax for a short time; then smear her face, and the backs of all the piglets, with a strong-smelling material—a kipper will often do. She will spend her time licking it off.

WHEN SOW IS SAVAGE

If the sow is particularly savage, then it may be necessary to call in your veterinary surgeon. It has been found possible by the use of modern anaesthetics or tranquillisers, to overcome such bad habits. When complete relaxation has taken place the litter can be placed alongside the dam, during which time they will suckle if left undisturbed. Light anaesthesia has the advantage over tranquillisers in that the effect, though adequate, is temporary, and when the dam recovers she will have forgotten her vicious intentions and will be unlikely to trample on her offspring as she might well do when under the influence of a tranquilliser.

If a sow starting to farrow shows signs of being nasty an injection of 1,500 i.u. PMS (pregnant mare's serum) should be given straight away—either during farrowing or immediately afterwards. The piglets are taken away and put in a container under an infra-red lamp for eight hours and hand-suckled. The litter is then quietly replaced.

A further and often overlooked cause of savaging is the presence of skin parasites. While lice are unlikely to be so extensive as to cause irritation, considerable pruritis or itching can be created by mange parasites. This causes unrest and frequently leads to bad temper and savaging (for control and treatment see section on mange).

If a sow is successfully restrained from eating her young, there is no reason why she should not be bred again. But where the sow has been guilty of cannibalism you must be particularly observant the next time she farrows, and see she has no opportunity to damage another litter. If she attempts to do this a second time, she should be fattened off. Possibly the pink appearance of the newly-arrived litter and the afterbirths may stimulate the urge, so afterbirths should be removed from sight as soon as possible. Within three or four days, not only have the piglets become whiter, but they are also more easily able to escape from danger.

TO ENSURE GOOD MILK FLOW

It is a good thing to cut the piglets' teeth. Should this not have been done and the milk flow is poor, the irritation and scratching caused by the teeth may well aggravate the sow, so that she loses her temper. To ensure a good milk flow and induce contentment, some workers have achieved success by giving 3 c.c. of pituitrin and 1 million units of penicillin, injected intramuscularly, the latter presumably to reduce the risks of mastitis.

If the sow is off colour or irritable for any reason, she may also be over-rough with some of her litter and do them harm.

Some sows are unduly cumbersome and careless and will not even be stirred by the squealing of their offspring.

TREATMENT AFTER FARROWING

Just a point here about treatment of the sow after farrowing. She will most likely welcome a drink. So give her either warmed cow's milk or warm water. A few hours later a warm bran mash or thin gruel 2 or 3 lb (0·90 or 1·35 kg) of wheat flour mixed with hot water and left to cool) should be offered.

This can be repeated night and morning for two or three days when, of course, cold water should be made available.

Solid food should not be given until 24 hours after farrowing; then only a moderate amount, followed by a gradual build-up to full rations a week after the event.

As a general guide, after 10 days the sow should be receiving 2 lb (90 g) meal daily for herself, plus 1 lb (450 g) of meal for each piglet. In any case she will take from 12-14 lb (5-6 kg). Adequate water should be available in a separate trough to ensure satisfactory milk yield.

Cutting the Teeth

Some farmers make a practice of nipping the youngsters' teeth before allowing them to suckle; others don't bother and apparently get no trouble.

It is largely a matter of choice. On the whole I favour doing it. It is a means of preventing teat and udder injuries that may cause the sow to withhold her milk. This will have an effect on the piglets' growth and may lead to mastitis in the sow.

Cutting the teeth is a simple job. The best instrument for this purpose is a strong pair of clippers such as are used for cutting dogs' claws. Clip the teeth close to the gums and remember that there are eight to cut—two top and two bottom each side. Cut by applying force and without any twisting (the job should, of course, be done out of the sow's hearing).

Care should be taken not to break them off, as germs may get into the gums causing infection and a lump on the jaw.

De-tailing

Removal of the tail within 12 hours of birth is the only sure way to combat the vice of tail-biting or chewing. Removal close to the root with a sharp scalpel is very effective and little or no bleeding occurs. Crushing the tail with a Burdizzo castrator is equally effective. Some people believe that it is advisable to leave a quarter to a third of the tail as it is only the bushy tip which seems to be most attractive to the aggressor.

Castration

This, of course, is a management matter and not a disease problem. Nevertheless a reference to the veterinary aspect will be helpful.

Castration of hog pigs is best done early, when they can be most readily caught and when the operation is likely to give the minimum of shock. Any time between 10 days to three weeks is suitable in this respect. There is also less bleeding. If attempted earlier some testicles may not be readily detected, and castration may not be so certain and a number of rig pigs may be left.

The operation requires some skill and experience, and due care should be taken as regards cleanliness and prevention of infection, otherwise an abscess may develop or lockjaw be produced (see page 131).

The pigs should be given a good bedding of clean straw three or four days before the operation to ensure that they are reasonably clean and not caked with muck. Clean bedding should be maintained after the operation too.

The operator should make a point of having clean hands. He should not handle the pigs but should leave that to an assistant.

STEP-BY-STEP PROCEDURE

The procedure will then be:

1. Catch the animal and hold it as shown in the photos between pages 80 and 81.

2. Clean the scrotum—the skin covering the testicles—with methylated spirits or a suitable non-sticky disinfectant.

3. Take a special castration knife or a new razor blade in a holder. See that the instrument is clean.

4. Cut down onto one testicle just deep enough to cut through the skin and the white membrane. Make an incision down the length of the testicle. The cut should be just long enough to let the testicle through easily—about 2 in (50 mm) is usually about right.

5. Pull testicle through the opening, twist twice and sever the cord with a scraping movement (a clean cut through will result in bleeding).

6. Repeat for the second testicle.

7. Dust into the cavities some antiseptic powder such as boracic acid or sulphanilamide.

Some people like to remove the testicles by pulling with a quick, vigorous movement instead of "scraping" through with a knife, but there is some risk of internal bleeding this way.

If there is a rupture and the bowel is protruding into the scrotal sac it is probably best not to castrate the animal yourself but to leave it to a veterinary surgeon. Although the swelling may become quite large, pigs seem to thrive quite well, but they should be slaughtered somewhat earlier than normal animals.

Animals need not be starved before castration if under seven weeks of age. Before you start the operation, however, be sure to remove the sow out of hearing. The squealing is not due to pain.

The use of rubber bands or bloodless castrators is not to be recommended as the testicles are not so clearly defined in their scrotum as in other animals and the risk of damaging the skin, and missing or only partially removing the testicles, is appreciable.

Artificial Rearing

It does occasionally happen that a sow or gilt dies at farrowing, or shortly after, leaving a litter of orphaned pigs to be reared. While it is possible to distribute a number of these piglets to other sows by using various subterfuges, such as smearing them with the afterbirth of the foster-sow, the development of satisfactory sowmilk substitutes has greatly simplified the rearing problem.

In an emergency, it may be necessary to rear the orphaned litter from birth. A proprietary milk substitute is then prepared in liquid form, according to the maker's recommendations, and fed in shallow troughs. On no account should piglets be forced to drink by pushing their heads in the troughs. It is better to encourage them by finger feeding or squirting a little of the fluid down the throat. If placed in troughs, piglets will frequently sip a little on their own accord and, finding it attractive, will quickly increase their intake.

The liquid should be provided fresh about every three hours for the first few days, the number of feeds being reduced and the concentration being increased as rapidly as possible, so that within five to seven days the substitute is being offered in dry form, either as powder or pellets. The sooner this stage is reached the better, as the risk of scouring on solid food is less than on liquid food.

No elaborate apparatus is necessary, but what is used should be simple, easy to sterilise and should be heavy enough to prevent spillage. Elaborate containers are not only unsuitable, but unnecessary and as it is not necessary to warm the milk, it will not go sour so readily.

A very suitable container for the dry feed is a large concrete brick with a deep frog. When a trough is introduced allow 6 in (150 mm) of feeding space per piglet, divided up into sections so that the piglets cannot stand in the trough. Until piglets have got thoroughly used to the dry powder place the water trough adjacent to the feed trough, but widen the distance a few inches (mm) each day, to reduce contamination of the food with drips from the water trough.

Early Weaning

In order to increase the number of litters per year and the rate of turnover of piglets, many farmers have introduced earlier weaning than the orthodox eight weeks. This has proved successful but cannot be pushed too far. Weaning at five weeks is practical and satisfactory. Weaning at three weeks is also effective though requiring more careful management. Shortening the period still more is not to be advised. As the suckling period is progressively shortened, so the sow takes longer to return to oestrus and litter numbers tend to fall. In cage rearing, however, where suckling for the colostrum is allowed for 4-7 days, there are advantages in the improved health of the litter, and the sow's food need not be reduced. But to ensure return to heat in good time, a boar should be run with the sows or be so placed that he can be smelt, heard and touched.

Piglets should be encouraged to grow as rapidly as possible by offering creep food. This may be provided as meal or pellets; either form is readily taken so long as it is fresh and highly palatable. A little white sugar or a few corn-flakes sprinkled on top or the use of a flavouring agent such as apple juice or chocolate flakes make creep foods very attractive.

At about 3–5 days of age small heaps should be placed on a clean piece of floor under the heat lamp. The frog of a brick makes a good 'trough'. Any surplus should be removed at night and a fresh supply put out daily until the piglets are really beginning to eat. In general, piglets seem to take readily to such substitutes especially in pellet form.

It is doubtful whether the feeding of milk substitutes will ever be more satisfactory than the sow's milk for the first three weeks of life, but undoubtedly litters reared artificially grow more rapidly as compared with those left on the sow during the latter half of the normal suckling period of eight weeks.

Incidentally, the composition of sow's milk (after the colostrum has gone) is: Total solids 15 per cent, fat 6·1 per cent, protein 5·4 per cent, sugar 5·9 per cent and ash 0·8 per cent.

Where artificial rearing is carried out either voluntarily or involuntarily, if the feeding methods are satisfactory they will not only give higher weaning weights, but will ensure, in general, more uniform and healthy litters than occur under the variable conditions of natural rearing.

When on sowmilk substitutes, either in liquid or porridge form, there is a tendency for the piglets to get coated with the food, the powder sticking to the nose and face, cheeks and ears. Sometimes quite hard crusts form, the skin becoming sore underneath.

If piglets are overcrowded, have insufficient trough space or get bored, they start to lick each other. This may lead to them chewing the ears and tails of their mates, and cannibalism may result. This risk can be reduced by mixing some barley meal, or some creep food, with the milk powder. Here the advantage of having the water and the food trough at least three feet (912 mm) apart will be appreciated.

Cage rearing from 7-10 days of age has certain advantages in that the conditions of stress which predispose to illness and losses during the first few weeks of life (fluctuating humidity, temperature and light, and competition for food) are avoided.

The Fading Piglet

Now come the disease problems likely to arise between farrowing and weaning. This used to be called "baby pig disease".

But there are many diseases of baby pigs, hence the more distinctive name to describe the condition.

When discussing this condition, we must be very careful to define it as there are a number of causes of mortality during the first few days of life and this is only one of them.

In a typical case, the litter is usually normal in size and appears healthy. The sow has adequate milk, yet within 24 to 48 hours of birth the piglets will lose interest in suckling and fall back. They begin to shiver and tend to wander away from the sow and hide under the straw. Up until this time they have appeared very healthy and have suckled well, a fact which is invariably confirmed at post-mortem by a full stomach.

Mortality may be 100 per cent and affect every litter born on a farm over a period of a few months after which it suddenly disappears.

The condition must not be confused with illness resulting when the sow has been slightly off colour or is suffering from low-grade mastitis or simple agalactia. But where piglets have been chilled and fail to suckle, due to unfavourable environment, the temperature and humidity of the farrowing pen may be an important factor and should be appropriately adjusted. Certainly fewer cases have been recorded since heated creeps became popular.

The fading pig syndrome is usually associated with a rapid fall in the blood sugar, the level of which is maintained temporarily by drawing on the liver reserves. Such reserves are naturally small in a new-born piglet and depend, in fact, on a continuous intake of milk. If milk is forcibly withheld from piglets, their blood sugar will fall very rapidly.

Why the piglets should suddenly become depressed and aimless is not known, although once the blood sugar begins to fall this is understandable.

The condition appears under different systems of management, though less in outdoor systems than others. The fact that the litter can be successfully reared artificially and independently of the sow, even after piglets have started dying, lends colour to the view that there is some deficiency in the sow's milk or that farrowing conditions are adverse. So one way of overcoming the problem is to take the piglets away and rear them artificially.

A treatment which has produced some success is the feeding of half-a-teaspoonful of 25 per cent glucose solution starting when the disease is suspected—a few hours after birth. Otherwise introduce the treatment as soon as possible and continue it every six hours for 24 hours.

Recent work has shown that the thyroids of such piglets are deficient in weight and structure, a situation which can be reproduced by exposing sows to cold, damp conditions for a few weeks before farrowing and during farrowing. There seems some justification from the evidence so far available for the addition of iodine to the sow's ration. This can be given at the rate of approximately 15 grams potassium iodide per ton of food for two or three months.

A final point—you need not have any fears about breeding the sow again. Although her milk is suspect when such a case occurs, the same trouble is not likely to arise after subsequent farrowings.

Haemolytic Disease or Baby Pig Jaundice

This peculiar disease has only been recognised of recent times. While there is no reason to believe that it is of great economic importance at the moment, it may be responsible for increasing losses in the future. In order to understand it properly, let us consider the phenomenon of what is known as antibody production in the blood.

When a foreign body such as a bacterium or a virus is present in the blood, it produces a stimulus which results in the development of so-called antibodies against the invading substances, and such blood will have the effect of suppressing or combining with the specific bacteria or viruses when put in contact with them.

Now, there are certain blood groups recognised in pigs, just as there are in human beings, and if a blood containing say an X group is injected into an animal, whose blood does not already carry the X group, it develops antibodies against that X group. If the latter blood is mixed later with a blood sample from an animal containing the X group, it will react with it and cause the destruction of the red blood cells. Moreover, the antibodies against this X group are secreted in the milk and can be conveyed to the piglet and absorbed into its blood. If the latter's blood contains this X group, then its blood cells are likewise pounced upon and destroyed, resulting in a reduction of the number of red cells, causing a paleness due to induced anaemia. In the course of destruction much pigment may be liberated into the blood, setting up a state of jaundice, so that the pigs appear with a yellow skin and membranes.

Whilst this state of affairs may happen under certain unknown circumstances, in practice it is likely to occur when animals lacking the X factor are injected with blood containing it, whereupon antibodies to X are developed. This situation was likely to arise when pigs were vaccinated with swine fever vaccine made from pig's blood (crystal violet vaccine).

If a boar with the X factor is mated to a sow lacking this factor, the piglets will receive the factor from the sire. When the sow is later vaccinated, the anti-X factors pass via the milk to the piglets and so into their blood, there reacting with the X group and causing serious symptoms or death, according to the degree of reaction. One injection of vaccine into the sow does not appear to have any serious effects, but two or more may, on occasion, precipitate the condition and cause heavy losses.

Piglets are born normal and suckle well, but in their first suck of milk take in the antibodies which pass through into their blood, and if conditions are appropriate, then their blood is affected and they show the above-mentioned symptoms.

There is no evidence that the disease can be responsible for stillbirths or deaths in the womb.

The disease is most likely to occur in litters from Saddleback sows, as Large Whites rarely produce these antibodies.

The body of an affected pig may become slightly yellow in colour, sometimes a muddy orange. This is the best recognition sign, although the colour change is sometimes difficult to notice in coloured pigs. It is best, therefore, to hold up the pigs by the hind legs and examine the skin of the belly and groin for any yellowish colouring.

Purpura

This is again a question of antagonistic blood factors, but it is the blood platelets not the red cells that are involved. It is similar to the rhesus problem in humans.

The boar has some factor in his platelets which the sow's platelets have not. The sow becomes sensitised through the leakage of some of the piglets' blood through the placenta during pregnancy, and when the piglets eventually suckle, the antibodies in the colostrum generated by the sow tend to destroy the piglets' platelets, so preventing clotting. This explains the purple blotches and lines seen under the thin belly, skin and ears shortly before death at about two weeks of age.

Anaemia

Anaemia can cause trouble up to weaning age. The first sign is generally a paling of the skin, especially around the ears and face. It is best described as paper-white. The paleness is not readily detected in black pigs, although a yellow tinge if present can usually be seen.

To understand the treatment and prevention of this disease it will help if we examine the cause.

After a piglet is born and starts to get its oxygen by breathing, it no longer requires the large number of red blood cells it needed to collect its oxygen when developing in the womb. So it begins to get rid of a lot of them.

A considerable reduction takes place during the first two or three weeks of life.

Even under proper rearing conditions the number of red cells actually falls below the optimum level, although this is a very temporary phase and is followed by a quick return to normal.

But where pigs are exposed to chilling or cold, damp conditions, or a shortage of minerals—especially iron, copper and cobalt—the loss of blood pigment continues and a state of anaemia becomes obvious.

It is a remarkable fact that the milk of the sow contains only one-fifteenth of the daily iron requirement of the piglet and it is not possible by feeding additional minerals to the sow, to raise the level in the milk. But specialised iron compounds are being tested which, when fed to the sow, will raise the iron level in the liver of the piglet whilst in the womb. Iron can also be picked up from the sow's dung. Mineral blocks are available but as intake is uncontrolled and there is increasing evidence that iron can be toxic, it is better to adopt a policy of injection where a controlled dose can be given.

The tenth day is critical. Scour, of a dirty grey or even a bright yellowish colour, develops.

Outdoor farrowing, or any system which permits the piglets to have an earth run and enables them to pick up their own minerals from the soil, is less likely to give rise to this disease.

ANTI-ANAEMIA MEASURES

The following anti-anaemia measures can be recommended:

1. If kept indoors put a shovelful of fresh earth taken from land which has not been over-run by pigs, into each pen daily. If soil is not available, then use a shovelful of cinders sprinkled with a copper and iron solution (half-a-gallon (2·27 l) of water and 1 oz (28 g) iron sulphate and $\frac{1}{4}$ oz (7 g) bluestone per 100 lb (45 kg) cinders). Use the cinders up to three weeks of age or until weaning, as required.

2. Another method of prevention is to give the piglets mineral tablets—containing cobalt and iron—when they are 24 hours old and repeat at the seventh and tenth day of age. These tablets can be obtained from your veterinary surgeon or chemist.

3. The application of an anti-anaemia paste (with a wooden spoon or spatula to the teeth or tongue) on the third, seventh and tenth days.

4. The injection of an anti-anaemia preparation between the third and seventh day is simple and successful and may be repeated according to the maker's instructions. This method is perhaps the most satisfactory, for it ensures that the piglet gets an adequate dose. Home treatment is, however, not to be

undertaken lightly. The use of a syringe is not all that simple, as indicated by the number of needles found in pigs' carcases at slaughterhouses.

As sub-clinical anaemia sometimes exists a second intramuscular injection at ten days of age is to be recommended as giving the maximum benefit in respect of the control of anaemia, improvement in growth rate and the reduction in cases of scouring.

It is probable that anaemia is not just a simple deficiency. Although it responds very well in most cases to the application of iron salts, the inclusion of B_{12} appears to have a beneficial effect. This is probably due to its known growth-stimulating properties. Indeed, I must stress that pigs kept in cold, damp conditions can still go down with anaemia, even if they are receiving preventive treatment or have access to soil. So warmth is the first essential in combating this disease.

Iron can be toxic, and where piglets receive no vitamin E in their dam's milk, symptoms of poisoning may arise.

Do not be too hasty to attribute scouring during the first few weeks to anaemia as there are many other causes which will be dealt with later. Post-mortem of pigs that have suffered from anaemia shows a pale, greatly enlarged heart.

Septic Toes and Knees

Sometimes little pigs are found to have gone lame on one foot and close examination will reveal that the coronet around one claw is swollen. It frequently overlaps the hoof and looks like a whitlow.

Occasionally there is a hole or sinus at the level of the coronet from which a slight discharge of pus exudes; sometimes the sole of the hoof has come off and is covered by a scab.

This condition usually arises because the bone in the hoof is diseased as a result of having been trodden on by the sow.

If the toe is amputated, the pig will go ahead immediately and will suffer no handicap. But if left in pain, several weeks may be required for recovery, during which time little growth will be made.

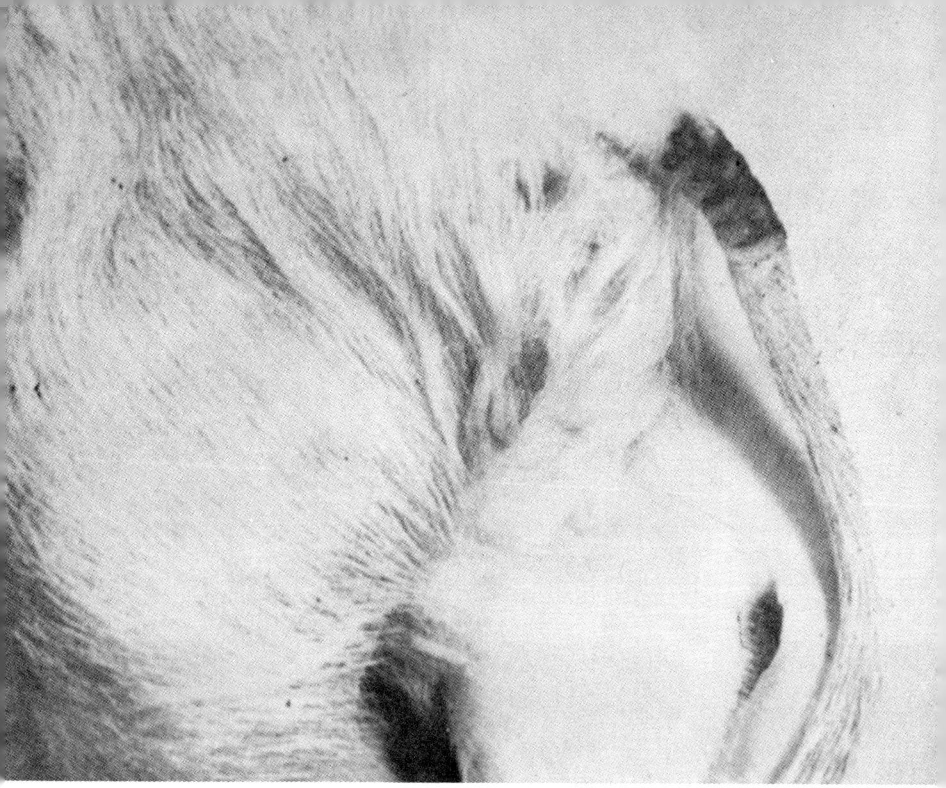

Ring tail—individual piglets often develop a scar on the tail after being trodden on or nipped. Necrosis or rotting may cause part of the tail to drop off.

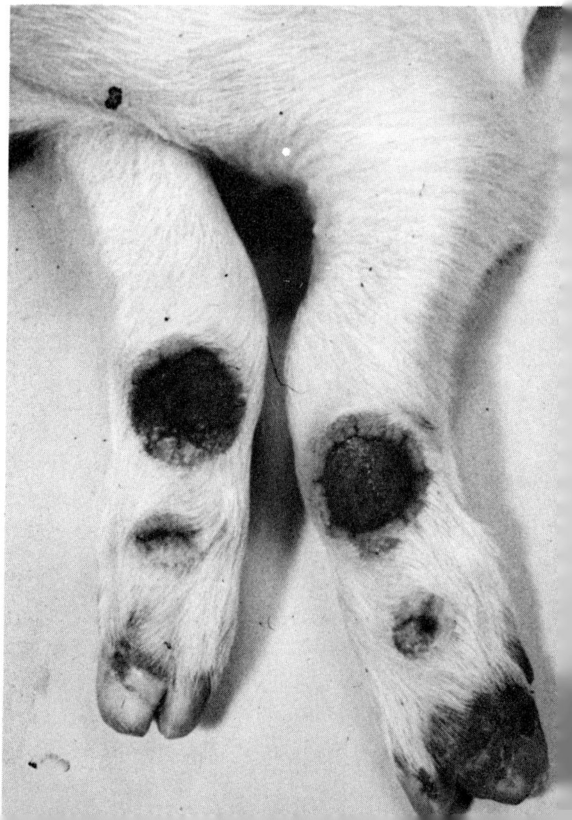

Scabby knees due to the creep floor being too rough are aggravated in large litters when the pigs have to compete for the sow's teats.

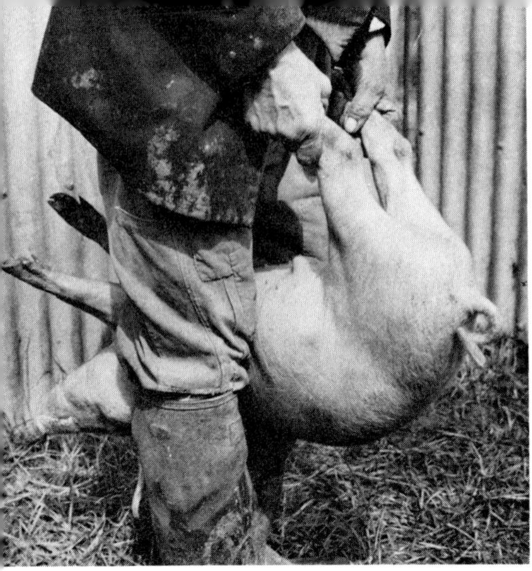

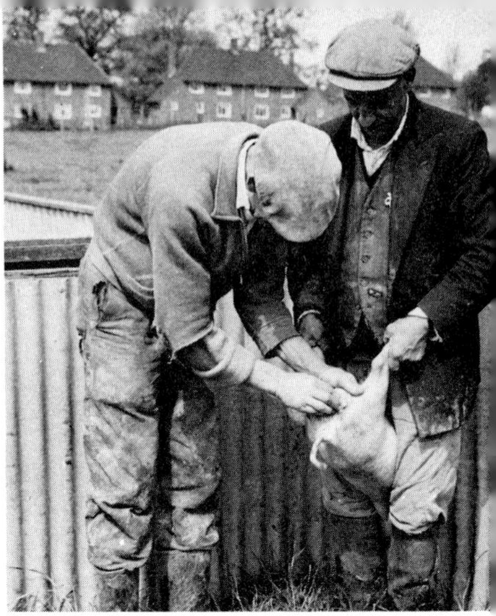

When castrating a pig grip its shoulders between your knees and hold its hind legs with a firm but relaxed grip.

When an assistant holds the pig firmly, you free to perform the operation quickly cleanly.

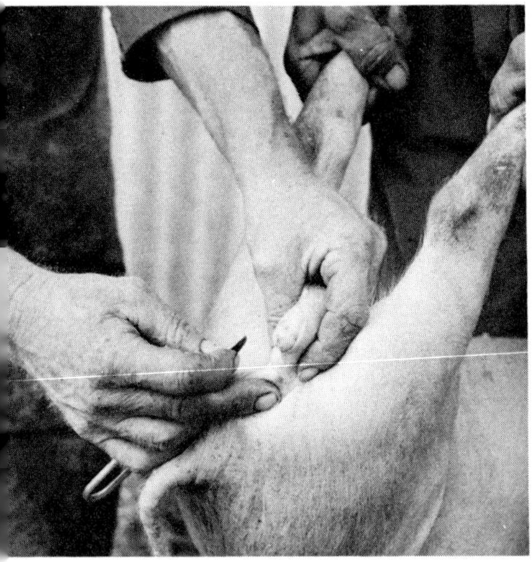

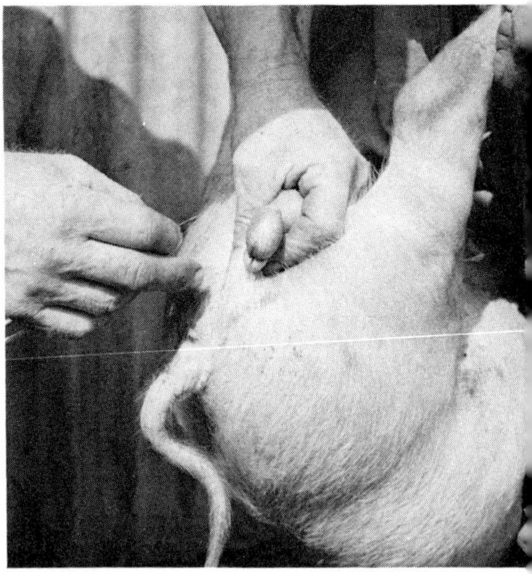

Above: Make a 25 mm cut in the base of the stretched scrotum, deep enough to penetrate the fairly thick layer of skin and the inner membrane enclosing the testicle.

Above right: If the testicle is held under pressure by the fingers behind it, and the cut has been made deep enough, the testicle will now pop out of the scrotum and can be pulled out on its cords.

Right: Instead of cutting the second cord, some pigmen prefer to pull it out at the roots.

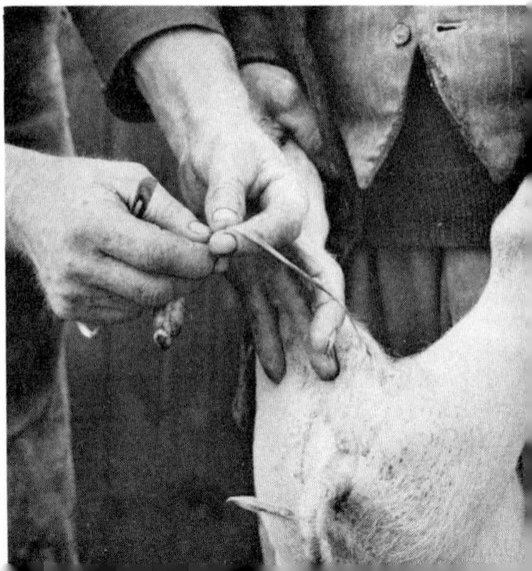

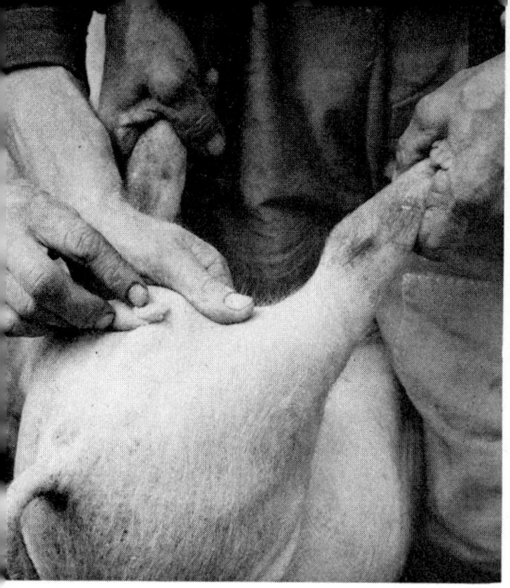

Clean the scrotum and surrounding skin with a mild antiseptic to prevent dirt and germs entering the wound.

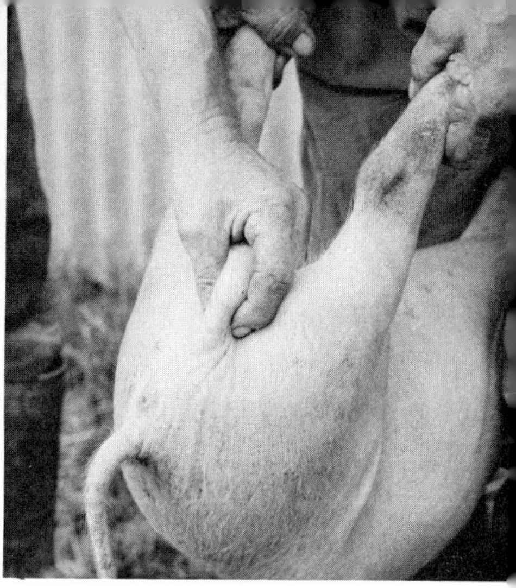

Grip one of the testicles firmly through the scrotum and press behind with the fingers to stretch the skin over it.

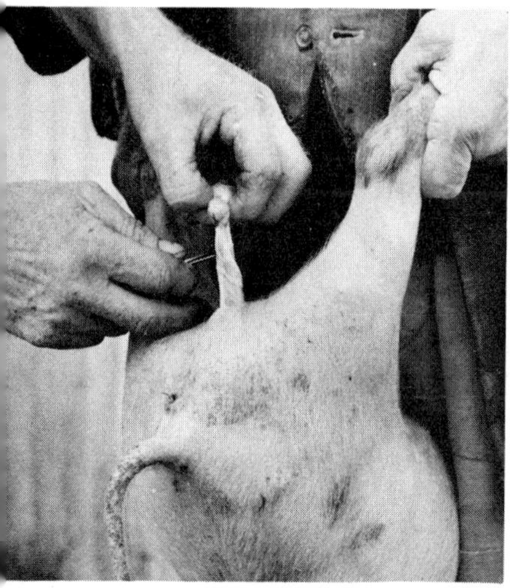

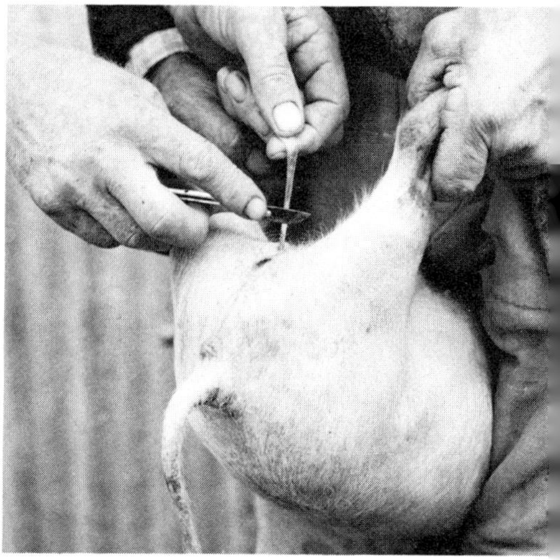

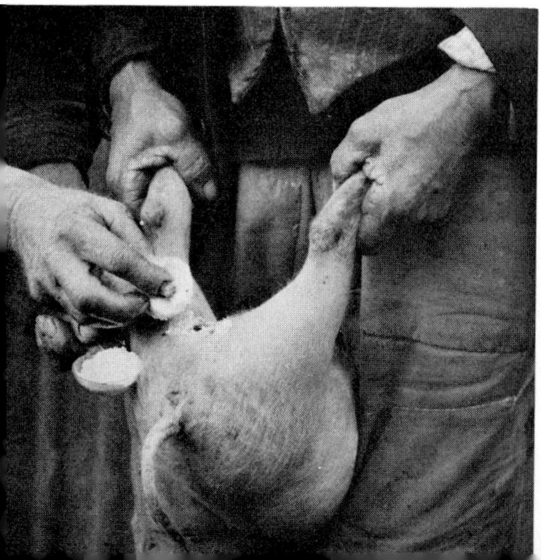

Above left: The testicle is attached by two distinct cords. Cut through the first, which looks like a white fatty membrane.

Above: The second cord is thinner, tube-like dark red in colour, and contains a vein. To prevent excessive bleeding scrape through this cord to make a jagged cut which will close and heal quickly.

Left: After removing the second testicle, dress the wound with antiseptic or sulphanilamide powder.

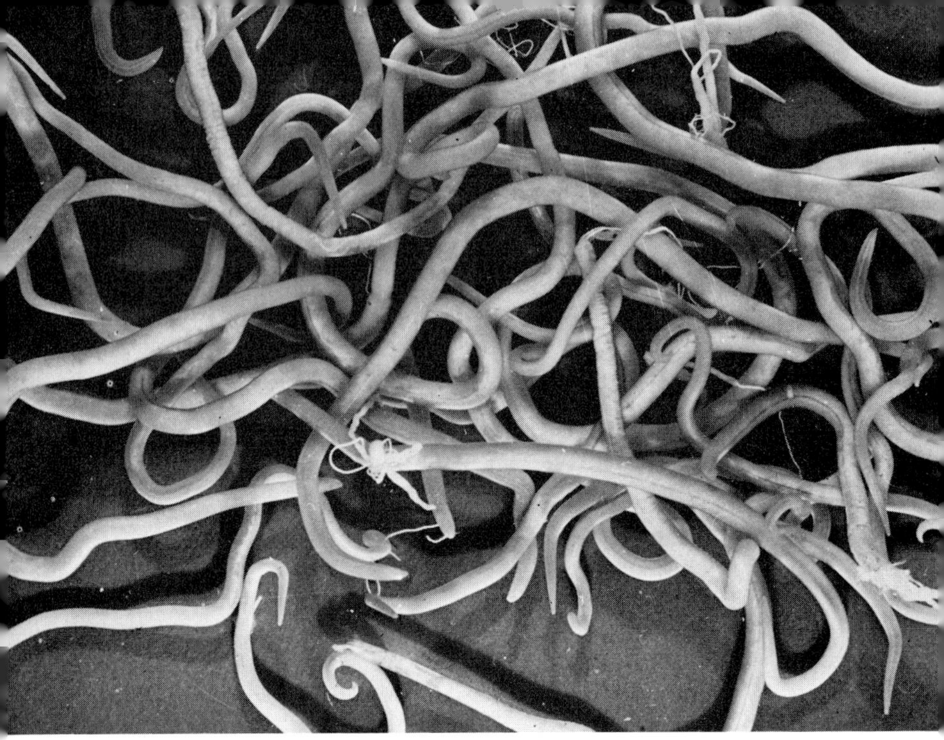

Large roundworms.

Photo: Boots Pure Drug Co. Ltd.

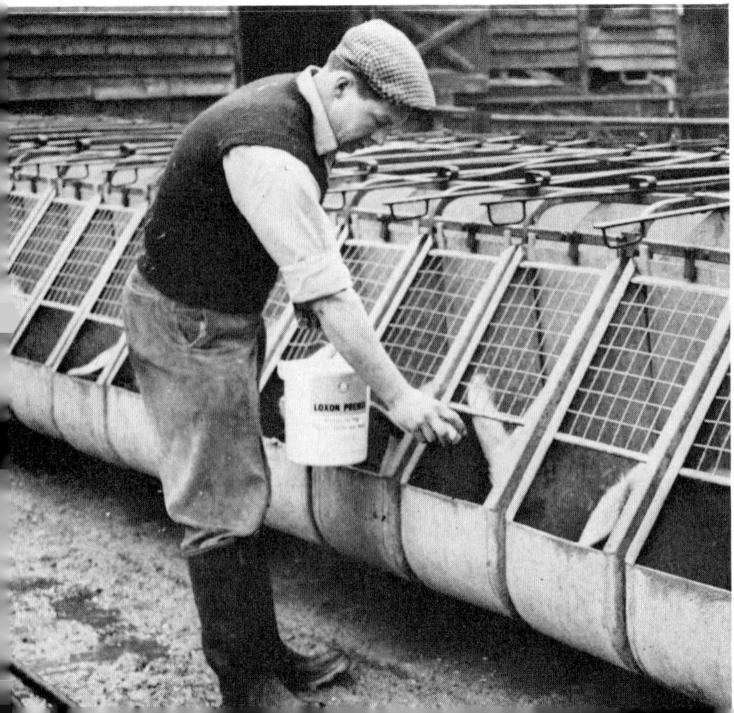

Feeding stalls ar useful when worm ing sows individu ally.

Photo: Cooper McDougall & Robertson Ltd.

Very often this condition is accompanied by sores on the knees of piglets, which have been produced as a result of struggling on a bare concrete floor when suckling. They generally recover spontaneously but if infection should penetrate and joints become affected, septicaemia may occur and an injection of sulphadimidine should be given.

The condition is common when milk flow is slow to start or remains poor, or there are not enough teats. Floors should be smooth and sawdust used as bedding.

Ring Tail (Necrosis)

Individual piglets up to weaning age often develop a scar somewhere on the tail. This is probably due to it being stepped on or nipped. Severe damage may lead to necrosis or rotting and a piece of the tail may fall off. Cases have, however, been encountered in which many piglets in many litters are affected. Obviously some more general cause is then operating. Ergot contamination of the sow's food could be responsible as the active principle of the ergot has the effect of constricting terminal blood vessels and so leading to necrosis of appendages.

Baby rats exposed to low temperatures have also been known to lose their tails, especially when the fat in the diet is poor in quality. The tail becomes bloodless because the vessels are constricted to keep blood within the body to conserve heat. It is possible that these observations have some bearing on the problem in pigs.

Arthritis

Lameness, together with swelling of the knee or hock joints (or both) can indicate a condition of arthritis. It may occur from about five weeks of age onwards. It is accompanied by high temperature and affected pigs will show signs of pain on movement or handling.

The condition can be cured if prompt action is taken. Veterinary treatment with sulpha drugs will do the trick; the sooner they are given the fewer doses will be necessary.

Repeated infection with erysipelas will also cause arthritis, but the condition can be largely controlled by the immediate use of erysipelas serum.

Since in older animals arthritis is frequently a result of similar repeated mild attacks or erysipelas, the use of erysipelas vaccine is to be recommended in any herd where the disease persists.

A type of acute septic arthritis (Glasser's disease), associated with streptococci, which causes lameness in young animals is quite common. Often in older animals a more chronic form associated with a stapylococcus is found. Whilst the former may affect several limbs, the latter is usually confined to one limb, causing a hot, painful, slightly swollen joint. Penicillin treatment is beneficial in the former and the sulpha drugs, including sulphamezathine, are to be recommended in the latter.

The SMEDI virus and mycoplasmas may also be responsible for arthritis.

Navel Bleeding

Though the cause of this condition is not known it could be hereditary. The litter is born normally and in some cases the cord may be red and swollen. Only a proportion of the litter is affected and there is a tendency for the cord to be broken off short or to be torn. If animals live for three days they will survive. Tests on blood show delayed clotting time which suggests there may also be nutritional factors involved. Perhaps there may be a deficiency, or an interference with the metabolism, of vitamin K.

Joint Ill or Navel Ill

Sometimes infection occurs through the navel at, or shortly after, birth. Various bacteria are concerned. An abscess may be formed at the umbilicus, or the bacteria may be conveyed in the blood-stream to different parts of the body.

The joints are often affected and a form of arthritis is common. There is marked lameness and affected pigs may die through being unable to suckle. Abscess formation may occur in various organs as well.

Every effort should be made to ensure that the navel is kept clean. If infection is suspected, douche with a reliable antiseptic and then dry it off with a powder. This can be either boric acid, iodoform or sulphanilamide. But too much interference can cause more harm than good. Do not cut the cord, but encourage it to dry off quickly. Naturally the best preventive measure, for all practical purposes, is a clean farrowing pen.

Observations suggest that in some cases, joint-ill is the result of an infection contracted either before birth or through the sow's milk. If the sow has become infected recently, she may not have had time to build up her resistance and pass protective antibodies in the milk to her litter.

The use of a mixed bacterial vaccine may help the sow to build up her resistance rapidly in these circumstances.

Aujeszky's Disease (or Mad Itch)

This is a disease particularly of young pigs of a few weeks old to two or three months of age. It is caused by a filterable virus which attacks the nervous system. Adults appear to be resistant and seldom show symptoms, though they sometimes abort and can develop pneumonia.

Though youngsters may not always show symptoms they usually stop suckling, become dull, shiver and develop muscular tremors. Subsequently they throw fits which increase in frequency. Each spasm may last for about a minute and then pass off, leaving the piglet exhausted. Death usually occurs during one of these fits. Mortality may reach 90 per cent.

There seems to be a marked skin irritation, for the animal rubs itself against local objects, pushing its snout and mouth against the wall or scratching itself. The temperature may reach 105°F (40°C).

There is no treatment for this condition. Pigs under six weeks of age usually die, those over 14 weeks live. The incubation period for the disease is from 7 to 10 days and it is probable that infection takes place by inhalation of the virus. This disease must be distinguished from the hereditary condition known as "trembles".

Cattle and sheep, as well as dogs and cats, are known to be

susceptible to the condition, although only in the first of these have cases been reported in this country up to date. So far only a few cases have been confirmed in Great Britain.

Teschen Disease

This condition, sometimes called infectious pig paralysis, or virus encephalomyelitis, is a specific infectious condition due to a virus. It has been recognised in most of the countries of continental Europe, and has of recent times been identified in Great Britain.

The virus is excreted in the faeces for many weeks after the initial infection, which can be spread widely on the farm without being recognised as pigs may not show any symptoms. This can be determined by blood examination from time to time.

The disease occurs in three stages associated with the spread of the virus from the digestive tract to the lymphatic system, then to the blood, and finally to the nervous system. The paralytic stage is, however, rarely reached.

Pigs of all ages, especially suckling or newly-weaned pigs and animals recently introduced to a herd, are most commonly attacked. Outbreaks occur throughout the year with a high incidence in winter and spring.

After the incubation period of 14-35 days has passed there is a brief period of fever followed by one of nervous irritability. Epileptiform fits and muscle tremors may be precipitated by sudden noises and hypersensitivity becomes apparent, animals being unwilling to submit to handling.

A paralytic stage may then appear overlapping the former. There is muscular paralysis with progressive stiffness and inco-ordination. Death may result from paralysis of the respiratory muscles.

A high proportion of clinically-affected pigs die within two weeks, the remainder recovering in 3-4 weeks. In older animals the disease usually takes a milder form.

Diagnosis can only be made by a laboratory examination of nervous tissue.

Treatment should not be introduced before a firm diagnosis

has been made by a laboratory. Considerable success has been achieved with the combined use of swine erysipelas serum and antibiotics, but the more recent development of a formalised and modified live vaccine is likely to be of greater value where the disease is tending to become established. It is most important to establish a diagnosis because of the similarity of the acute form of this disease to swine fever.

Congenital Splay Leg (Myofibrillar Hypoplasia)

Litters born of Landrace parents not infrequently show a striking weakness of the legs and are unable to stand from birth. It is also occasionally seen in association with other breeds.

Within a few hours of birth the piglets endeavour to raise themselves, but are only able to stand on their forelegs. Some are able to drag themselves around and may be able to suckle. If they do, then they generally recover—the others which are unable to do so are likely to die. Whilst it has been suspected that this may be a nutritional deficiency—possibly of a member of the vitamin E or B complex—nevertheless, ready response occurs only when the piglets are assisted to suckle by moving them to their dam, and furthermore the condition is seldom reported in association with other breeds of pig, which suggests an hereditary weakness.

Research has shown that the muscle tissue is immature at birth, development of muscle fibres being incomplete. The situation is aggravated by the unusually long loin of the Landrace breed, but recovery occurs in two to three weeks if suckling is maintained.

Conditions Believed to be Inherited

As a conclusion to this chapter it is well to draw attention to a number of abnormalities believed to be inherited conditions and not problems of disease.

Hereditary defects occur when there is a failure in the reproduction process so that a variant or abnormal form is produced. This is known as a mutation, and mutants may be either dominant or recessive. If dominant, the defects can be immediately detected and eliminated. On the other hand, recessives cannot be spotted by inspection; breeding tests are necessary to identify them.

The following recessives are of a harmful nature and are referred to as lethals:

Imperforate anus (lack of back passage); piglets born alive.

Cleft palate (split roof to the mouth); leads to inability to suckle: born alive.

Water on the brain; sometimes stillborn.

Harelip; born alive.

Brain hernia (skull open); born alive.

Thickened forelimbs (due to connective tissue infiltration of muscle fibres); born alive.

Front and hind legs missing; born alive.

Paralysis (hind legs stiff); born alive.

Stiff or bent front legs; stillborn.

Split ears (associated with deformed hindquarters); stillborn.

Degeneration of the foetus in the womb.

Non-lethal factors that may be inherited are numerous; some examples are:

Trembles (characterised by violent shivering from two days to six weeks of age). There is no treatment; spontaneous recovery occurs towards the end of the suckling period. As this condition is harmless, the same mating may be repeated, though in 12-15 per cent of cases it has been found to be associated with swine fever, and was at one time a notifiable condition.

Hermaphroditism (occurrence of male and female genitals).

Scrotal hernia. This can be sewn up by a veterinary surgeon at the time of castration, if the pigs are castrated not earlier than six weeks of age.

Navel or umbilical hernia. This is difficult to treat; strangulation and peritonitis often secondary.

Blindness. There is some evidence that a dominant is involved, but the condition may also be due to lack of vitamin A.

Malformation of jaw (too short or too long lower jaw).

Failure of one testicle to descend.

Absence of certain parts of the genital tract in the female.

Inverted nipples may occur in a high proportion of females among one or more litters in a herd. These are flat to the touch, but not all teats are affected. The occurrence in a herd may be repeated with the same matings so it is better to dispose of the boar. With a good gilt it is worth massaging the teats with olive oil, as many will revert.

Pityriasis—a skin disease of variable extent lasting from 1–8 weeks in pigs under 12 weeks of age.

Other non-lethals are—kinky tail, hairlessness and sterility.

Where any of these defects occur in several pigs, and especially if they are repeated in subsequent matings, then the breeding should be investigated and one of the partners changed.

Prolapsed Rectum

Although prolapsed rectum is usually regarded as an hereditary weakness and can be stamped out by changing the boar, conditions associated with inflammation of the bowels, such as coccidiosis and other forms of acute enteritis, may be responsible for severe straining and eversion of the back passage. Before blaming the boar or dam, therefore, ascertain that there is no enteritis, or if there is, treat it first.

Where there appears to be no obvious cause, see that there is plenty of water available at a low level so that piglets have not got to stand up and strain to get it. Give each piglet a large dose of liquid paraffin and, at the same time, apply this with the finger up the rectum. It is often possible in the early stages to reduce a mild prolapse by applying the liquid paraffin as indicated, and stitching lightly across the rectal orifice. But where the rectal wall is very thin as when the hereditary defect occurs in Large Whites, an operation must be quickly done.

Vomiting and Wasting Disease

This condition affects young pigs up to four weeks of age and was first reported in Canada in 1958. There is first loss of appetite, then vomiting, and in a few days the faeces become hard and pelleted. There is progressive loss of flesh causing marked emaciation followed by death.

Encephalitis may also occur or be present by itself. Outbreaks of this form were reported in Ontario in 1962 and the disease was identified in the UK in 1969 when a virus resembling in some ways that of TGE was isolated and identified.

Mortality may be as high as 90 per cent and from the examination of sows' blood taken over a wide area it would seem that the distribution of the virus is widespread and infection often occurs without symptoms.

Chapter 6

DISEASES AND DISORDERS DUE TO FEEDING

THE previous chapter dealt with problems specifically relating to young pigs up to weaning age. The rest of this book will deal with troubles that are likely to occur at any time in a pig's life, but usually after weaning.

This chapter is concerned with diseases and disorders that are believed to be of nutritional origin.

We will deal with vitamin deficiencies first.

Vitamin A Deficiency

Where pigs are kept out-of-doors and have access to green food—especially grass—there should be no shortage of vitamin A, though the quality deteriorates in winter when rations need supplementing. The carotene present in the herbage is converted in the bowel wall to vitamin A and then stored mainly in the liver for further use.

But for indoor pig-keeping it must be remembered that a piglet is born with very low vitamin A reserves and depends upon colostrum to boost its initial supply. Thus it is important that the sow's ration should be adequately fortified in this respect.

Deficiency of maternal vitamin A, which is commoner in gilts than sows, can result in serious losses associated with full-time dead piglets. In the most severe form piglets are stillborn or die shortly after birth. Some piglets are undeveloped, and some show "water belly", or ascites. Those that are alive show no interest in suckling. None has the strength to walk normally, many of them lying on their sides gently paddling and squealing, making a sound which is quite characteristic of the condition. There is occasionally an accumulation of fluid under the skin giving the piglets a rounded appearance. In many cases the lids are glued together and the eyeballs rudimentary.

Abortions may occur and, in some instances, piglets are re-absorbed. In less severe conditions there are gross eye defects, and in the milder case it is again the eyes that are affected, but only slightly, associated with the position and extent of the iris. These litters could be reared but in some cases nervous symptoms and paralysis develop later.

A bare minimum of vitamin A may result in retardation of growth, and in a short time the head becomes unusually large in proportion to the body. Pigs look pot-bellied, the skin being spread tightly over the body. Stiffness of the legs develops and animals tend to walk on their toes. Appetite is not at first reduced—but later becomes poor; pigs become lethargic and tend to sit about in a dog-like attitude.

In sows where growth has ceased the symptoms may not be so striking, but heat periods may be prolonged, erratic or absent and subsequently convulsions may occur. The head may be held on one side and breathing become exaggerated.

Inflammation of the bowels and pneumonia are commonly revealed at post-mortem, although if killed in the early stages there is usually nothing to be seen.

When scouring is severe as in cases of enteritis, where there is a heavy worm burden, or in cases of pneumonia, vitamin A reserves are quickly used up, and even the incoming vitamin in the food may be insufficient in the circumstances. Moreover, the inflammation of the bowel may tend to interfere with the conversion of the carotene to vitamin A so exaggerating the condition. In such circumstances an injection of 100,000 units of vitamin A intramuscularly will materially benefit the animal. Green food, such as kale, silage, grass, and the legumes are high in carotene which as already mentioned is the precursor of vitamin A.

Vitamin B Deficiencies

There are a number of vitamins which constitute what is known as the vitamin B complex and, within this group, several different factors. As they frequently occur together in the same feedingstuffs in varying quantities, it is seldom that an obvious case of a single vitamin B deficiency is encountered.

The vitamins to be considered are:

Thiamin (aneurin B_1), Riboflavin (lactoflavin B_2), Biotin, Nicotinic acid, Pantothenic acid, Pyridoxine (B_6), and Vitamin B_{12}.

Below are the effects of deficiencies, as far as we know them.

Thiamin: Symptoms are obscure and include loss of appetite and retarded growth. The vitamin may be administered by injection or by mouth (see also bracken poisoning).

Riboflavin: A deficiency of this vitamin has not so far been shown to have any adverse effect, but its use in baby pig disease has been recommended.

Biotin: A deficiency causes loss of hair, dermatitis, shallow mouth ulcers and furring of mouth and oesophagus. Soft, cracked hooves are common. Vertical and in particular horizontal, reddish scars are seen, or square plaques on the lower edge of the hoof. The time from weaning to first heat may be prolonged. Supplementation improves matters and may give another piglet per litter.

Biotin occurs naturally, *e.g.*, soya, fishmeal, skim milk but is not fully available to the animal. Of 420 mc/kg in fishmeal only 25-50% is available. Grass is a good source.

Nicotinic Acid: This is likely to occur on a diet particularly high in maize. The lack of this vitamin results in stunted growth and progressive unthriftiness of young piglets associated with a marked enteritis and early diarrhoea. Symptoms resemble necrotic enteritis or "paratyphoid".

The condition clears up quite well on administration of the vitamin. Give affected pigs half-an-ounce (14 g) of dried bakers' yeast daily in their rations for about a fortnight and see that their ration contains good-quality animal protein which ensures the full utilisation of the nicotinic acid.

If suckling pigs are affected, give the yeast to the sow—at the rate of 2 lb per 100 lb (900 g per 45 kg) of food—for a fortnight.

Pantothenic Acid Deficiency: This is characterised in the young pig by watery diarrhoea leading to dysentery. Growth is impaired and there is a loss of hair. A cough may develop and nasal secretion become marked.

In a very limited number of cases a skin rash appears on the face, covering most of the face of the piglet a few days after birth and increasing in intensity up to four to five weeks of age after which it disappears spontaneously. If not attributed directly to a pantothenic acid deficiency, it is suggested that it is associated with a deficiency of one of the vitamin B vitamins in the milk, this view being reinforced by the rapid response to the use of Marmite pasted on the tongue.

It is nevertheless difficult to explain this condition on a deficiency basis as only a few litters out of a large number are generally affected from a bunch of animals all being fed on the same diet.

In recently-weaned pigs there may be unsteady gait, a gawky movement, with, later, twisted legs. Animals nevertheless eat well and remain alert, although there may be some scour and loss of condition.

In older animals the action of the hind legs is often abnormal and may become so striking that it resembles goose-stepping. There is also poor growth, loss of appetite, lachrymation, and there may be some dermatitis and scouring.

A deficiency may occur when the ration contains a high proportion of barley meal but this is only because the rest of the ration may be 'diluted'. There is not enough pantothenic acid in the barley alone. Good sources of appropriate vitamins are fish meal, liver meal, dried milk and brewers' grains, and, in an emergency, dosing with 500 to 750 milligrams of pantothenic acid daily for three or four days is effective. A minimum of 6-10 mg per pound (454 g) of food is desirable.

The animal usually rests on its buttocks and moves with considerable difficulty. When encouraged to do so it lifts the hind legs in an exaggerated fashion, swaying its rump sideways each time a leg is lifted. It quickly comes to rest and obviously prefers to remain lying down.

Pyridoxine: In its absence diarrhoea and unthriftiness occur. There is loss of appetite and occasional vomiting. There is nervous derangement with some staggering. The absence of this vitamin or the previous one may cause quite characteristic skin sores on the face which appear as irregular, warty growths of a dark colour. If a teaspoonful of Marmite is scraped on the tongue on several successive days, these sores rapidly disappear. Yeast is equally beneficial given at the rate of one ounce (28 g) of brewers' yeast per day.

Vitamin B_{12}: This vitamin has come into importance of recent times in relation to anaemia. It is now accepted as an essential growth factor which is, in the ruminant animal, manufactured in the rumen by certain bacteria that need cobalt for their multiplication. It is to be found in the animal protein part of feedingstuffs and may in fact comprise a large proportion of the so-called animal protein factor. While it is normally present in properly-blended rations containing materials of animal origin, such as fish meal, meat-and-bone meal and liver meal, it does appear to have a general growth-promoting quality. No condition of vitamin B_{12} deficiency has, however, as yet been clearly recognised in the pig.

Cereal foods are generally rich in vitamins of the B complex, but either brewers' or bakers' yeast contain such a high content of some of these that they are frequently used as a supplement.

Vitamin D Deficiency

This vitamin is associated with bone development and is obtained naturally by the animal by exposure to sunlight and, artificially by the feeding of cod-liver oil or synthetic vitamins.

In the presence of this vitamin bone formation develops

normally so long as the calcium and the phosphorus are present in the appropriate proportions. Should the ratio of calcium to phosphorus be too wide one way or the other, then symptoms of rickets may appear. Such symptoms have been precipitated by the heavy feeding of yeast, which is high in phosphorus, thus upsetting the ratio. But the modest supplementation of a few ounces (50-80 g) per pig per day that I have recommended in this book from time to time, for certain conditions, is unlikely to have any adverse effect in this respect.

If bone formation is interfered with in the growing pig and minerals are not being deposited properly, the bones remain rather soft and bend under the weight of the animal, becoming distorted in various ways. The ends of the bones become swollen though the shaft remains slender.

A characteristic of rickets is the "knobbing" of the rib joints, which can best be seen from the inside when the animal has been killed. This form of rickets is not difficult to diagnose and an adjustment of the ration will generally bring about marked improvement in the remainder, though the skeleton may still remain malformed.

In fattening pigs on a deficient diet, or one made so by feeding too much swill, pigs quickly become unthrifty, stand about with a humped back and a straight tail. There are signs of scouring and the pig eventually finds it painful to stand on its stiff joints. It quickly responds to good feeding.

Rickets frequently occurs in animals approaching breeding age. It first reveals itself as a slight stiffness—the animal becomes crampy and moves with great reluctance. When forced to do so by prodding it squeals loudly, but after a short spell of activity it seems to improve. There is no evidence of swelling of the joints and pain is only evinced as indicated above. The condition steadily gets worse. An injection of 10,000 to 20,000 units of vitamin D, repeated if necessary, generally brings about marked improvement.

This form of rickets must not be confused with the lameness and crampiness associated with swollen, painful joints caused by bacterial infection (see page 82).

Vitamin E Deficiency

Simple muscular dystrophy with pale striped "fish muscle" as in the calf is not characteristic of a deficiency of vitamin E in the pig. This fact and the possible masking or at least complicating effect of selenium in this context has made diagnosis more difficult. Mounting experience and increasing interest have, however, recently widened the field and if the situation has not been made simpler at least there is a greater awareness of the factors involved.

Treatment: It is all important that the ration should be adequate in vitamin E and this may need to be added as a standard ingredient in the future. Sows' rations must contain it if they are to behave normally themselves and pass on some to their offspring.

Piglets receiving no vitamin E in their colostrum appear to have an increased sensitivity to iron injections. The vitamin is also necessary for normal muscle growth and action.

As the sparing effect of selenium is now well established it may also be desirable to inject pigs with selenium in appropriate cases. The dose is extremely small, being in the region of 1 mg, yet there may be danger of toxicity if this is increased threefold. As the piglet grows however, its requirements will increase so that the available selenium will soon be inadequate and the second injection may be desirable at about three months to carry it on to bacon-weight.

There is evidence to suggest that vitamin E deficiency in the pig is not so rare as was hitherto believed, probably because of the difficulty of diagnosis.

Post-mortem changes reveal evidence of pale, striped muscle indicative of muscular dystrophy.

There is really no need for such vitamin deficiencies to occur with our modern knowledge of feeding and management. It is far better to avoid them by keeping animals on an adequate diet under satisfactory hygienic conditions than to have to attempt to cure them by subsequent treatments. However, 500 milligrams of alpha-tocopheryl acetate given daily for a week, should bring about a marked improvement when cases arise.

It is possible that the heavy feeding of grain (barley), harvested wet, may predispose or induce dystrophy in which case response to 2·5 mg of alpha-tocopheryl acetate and 0·01 mg of selenium per lb ($\frac{1}{2}$ kg) bodyweight is effective.

A condition associated with the sudden death of store animals subject to the strain of being carried to the market has been known for some time. Post-mortem reveals abnormal changes in the heart and this could be associated with a vitamin E deficiency, for this vitamin is very necessary for the nutriment and normal functioning of muscle tissue, especially that of the heart. Transit stress can be greatly reduced by giving 1 mg of Azerperone intramuscularly per lb ($\frac{1}{2}$ kg) bodyweight.

Hepatosis Dietetica

The above heading implies liver damage of nutritional origin, but the situation is complicated. The liver is enlarged, pale in colour and may show necrotic areas and haemorrhages. Vitamin E and the mineral selenium appear to work in harness and if one is absent the other can partially compensate for the deficiency. This would explain the small proportion of failures which follow the use of vitamin E by mouth. Selenium can also be given in liquid form or as an injection.

Mulberry Heart Disease

Cases of sudden death due to circulatory failure associated with a defective heart are recorded from time to time. In such cases the heart is irregularly swollen and congested and shows haemorrhages beneath the surface. Its superficial appearance suggests that of a mulberry.

Whilst the cause of the condition still remains obscure, there is increasing evidence to justify linking it with *Hepatosis dietetica.* It also resembles the German disease known as hertzod which merely means "dead heart"—again an abnormal heart associated with sudden death. Widespread congestion and haemorrhage is a constant finding in mulberry heart disease, although the abnormal areas in the heart in hertzod are pale greyish white or greyish yellow.

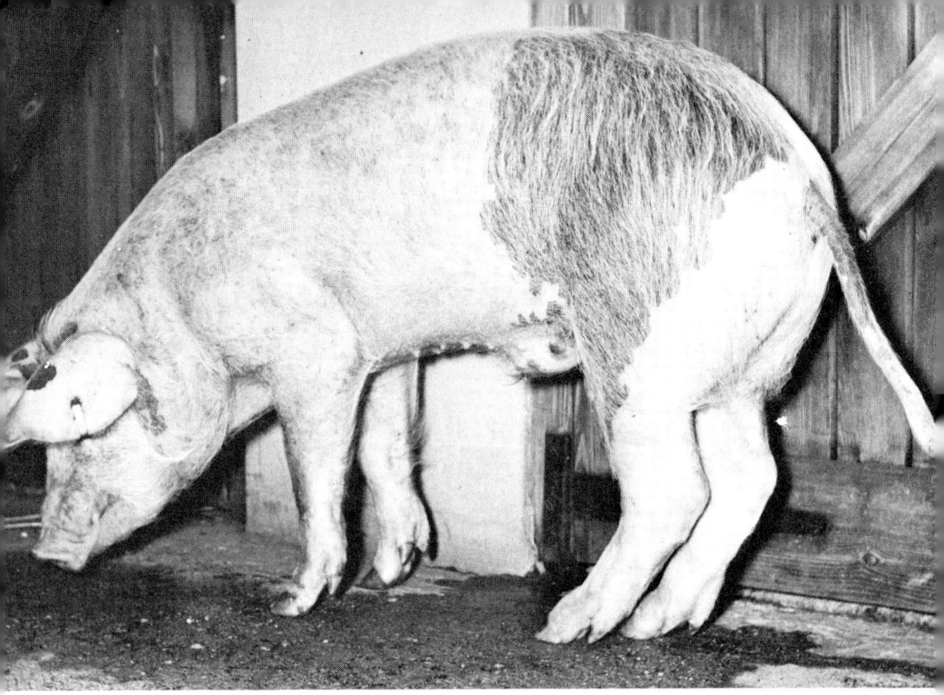

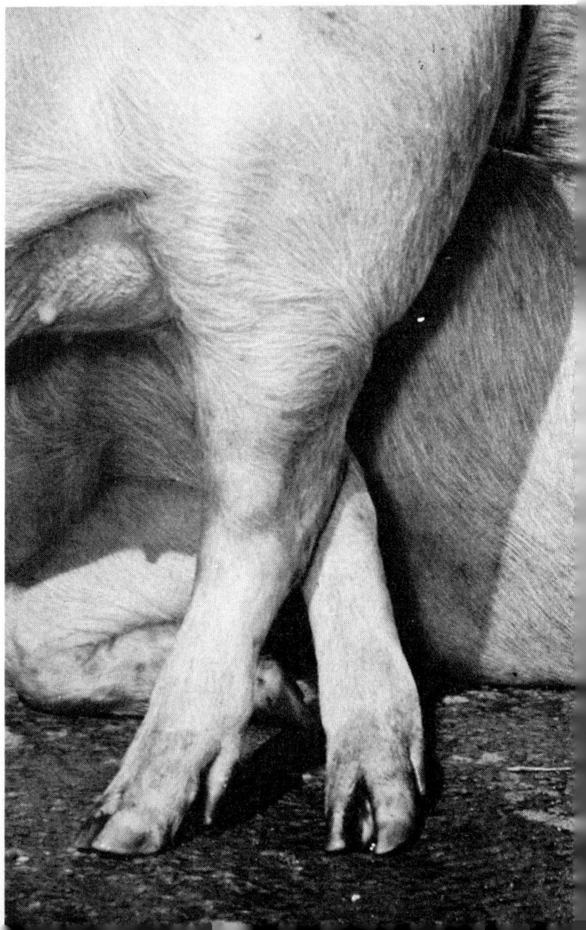

Pigs suffering from swine fever often have a swaying gait (right); their tails may be straight, too (above).

Clipping

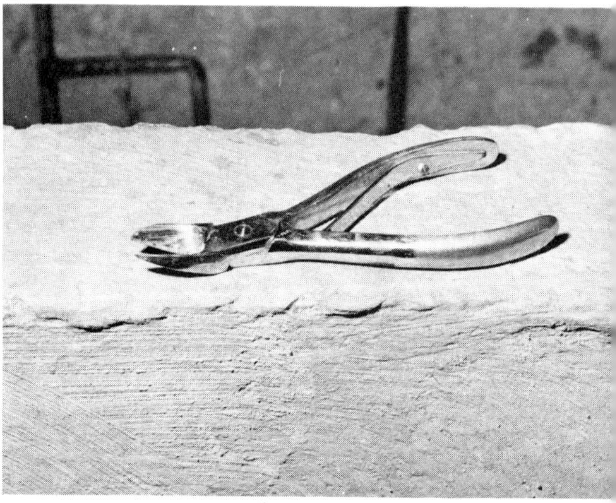

Cutting edges of these stainless-steel cutters are flat on one side and bevelled on the other. Before the operation cutters should be wiped clean with surgical spirit.

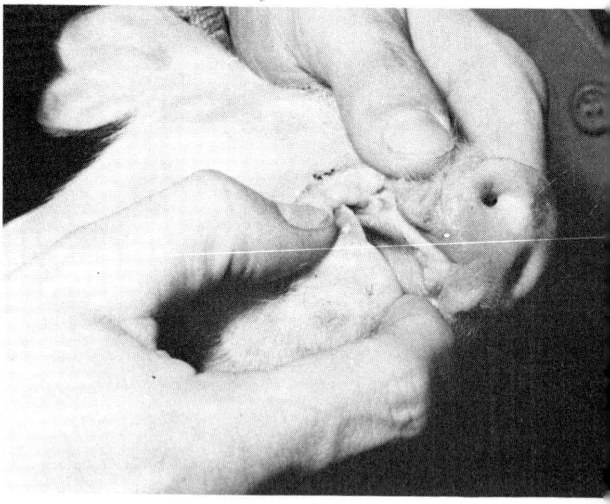

Prise open piglet's mouth with thumb and forefinger.

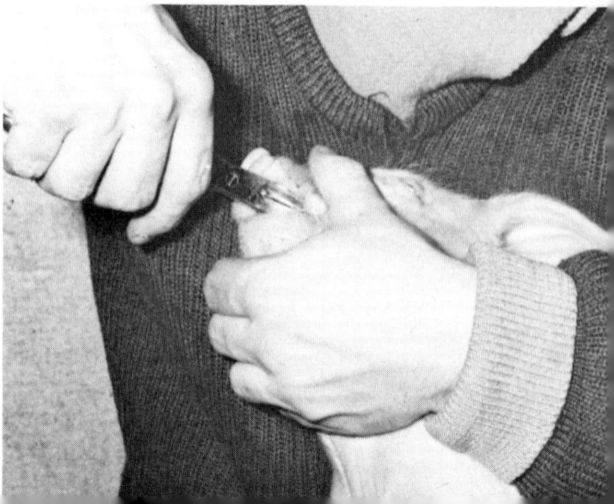

Insert clippers into the mouth from the front. Keep flat side of blades close to the gum, but take care not to cut it or the tongue. Clip the teeth cleanly without twisting or pulling.

let's teeth

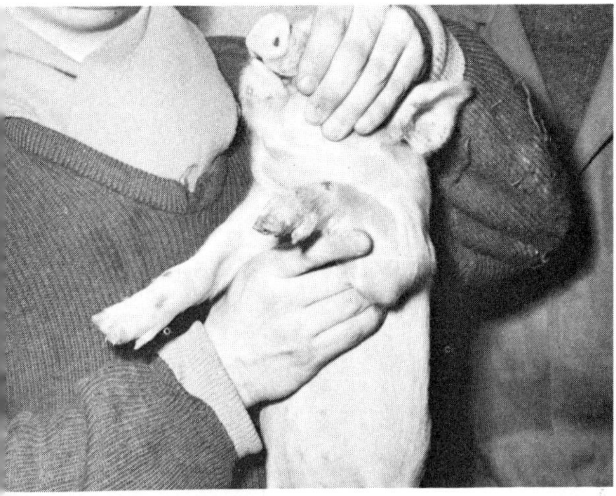

Best age to cut piglet's teeth is at a day old (this pig is older). There are eight teeth to be clipped—two at the top and two at the bottom of each side of the jaw.

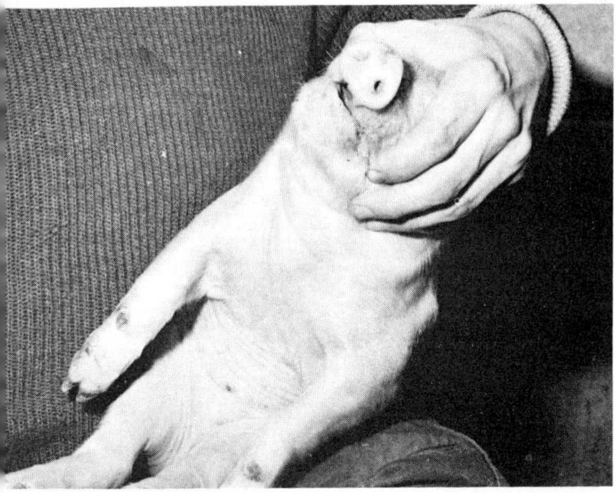

Support piglet on your thigh while keeping its mouth open.

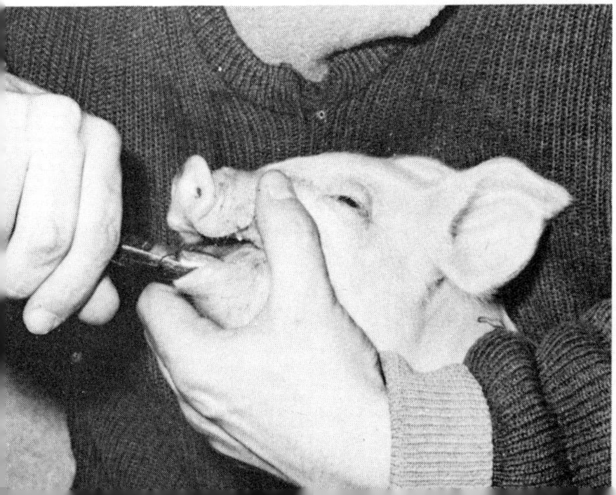

Don't forget to do the ones at the bottom. Then run your finger inside the piglet's mouth to see if there are any needle-sharp edges left.

Right:
Pityriasis rosea can cause a bran-like scaliness of the skin.

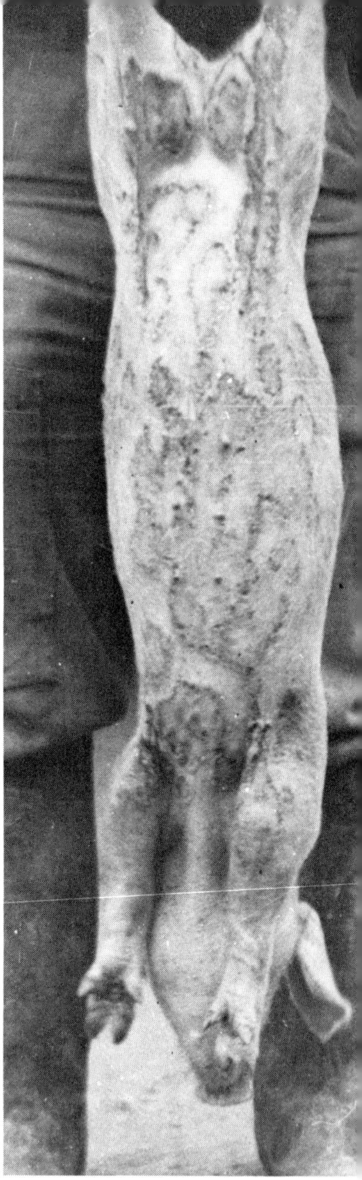

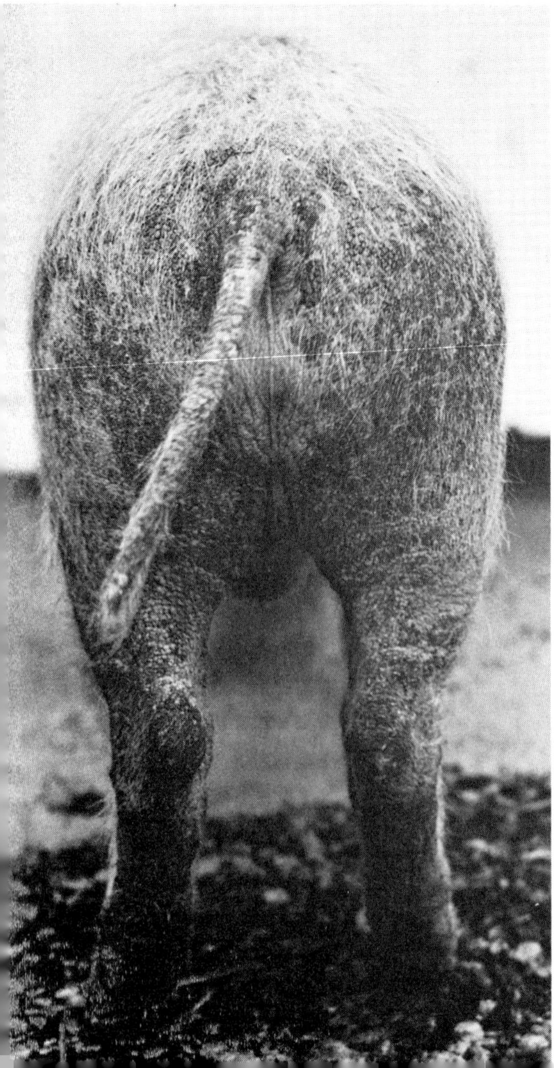

Left:
Parakeratosis (dirty skin disease) is due to lack of zinc in the pig's diet.

Haemorrhagic Scours

A very acute, bloody scour can sometimes be met with in pigs of about 80-100 lb (36-45 kg), and thriving well. They come up to the trough when this is filled but eat very little. At the next mealtime they will rush to the trough but fall over and die very quickly.

Post-mortem reveals marked haemorrhage into the bowels and blood splashings on the heart muscles. This condition, though rare, is usually associated with the feeding of grain which has been stored wet and become mouldy. In these circumstances the oxidation that has taken place could have destroyed the vitamin E, but the deaths are so sudden that a mould toxin cannot be ruled out. The rations should be immediately supplemented with vitamin E at the rate of 500-1,000 milligrams per pig daily for several weeks and the grain destroyed or used in very small quantities at a time for other purposes.

Whey Bloat and Gastric Torsion

Intestinal haemorrhage not infrequently occurs due to torsion and twisting of the stomach or intestines, so shutting off blood supply and causing rupture of blood vessels. Pigs fed whey sometimes develop *bloody gut*. Death is sudden, the carcase is pale and the abdomen distended. Post-mortem will show that the large and small bowels have been rotated, often by 180° round the suspending membrane (the mesentery). It is likely that the large volume of fluid associated with the fermentation of lactose and gas formation are predisposing factors in causing instability. The same could apply in the case of *gastric torsion* where it is the stomach that becomes twisted. However, the latter does not necessarily occur on whey feeding, though disproportionate distension of stomach or bowels is probably a basic cause.

Once-a-day feeding leading to excitement, an eager appetite and greedy feeding where there is competition, and especially when food is given in liquid form, are likely factors involved. The above conditions may well explain the syndrome previously described in this book as "White Pig Disease", in which the first indication of trouble is a marked pallor of the skin rapidly becoming accentuated in association with increasing internal haemorrhage; at the same time the droppings becoming brownish due to decomposed blood, death occurring 24 hours after the appearance of the first symptoms.

Stomach Ulcers

The previous section records the author's personal experience in the early 1960s. It was not until 1970 that cases were first recorded in the UK.

Feeding experiments have suggested that rations containing finely ground maize appear to encourage ulceration, whereas in one experiment 50 per cent only were affected on a wheat-oats based ration. No ulcers occurred on an all-oats ration.

It is difficult to explain the protective effect of oats (and to a less extent wheat), but when considering the consistency of rations, it seems clear that where ulcers occur, the stomach contents have usually been markedly fluid as distinct from the more solid mass found in normal stomachs. Acid secretion may sometimes be increased but not in every case. Mechanical irritation can be ruled out since coarse sand, even up to 50 per cent of the ration, appears to have no ill effect other than to suppress appetite. A coarse-ground ration is far less likely to cause ulcers than a very finely ground one.

Over-crowding and other stress factors, whilst not initiating ulcers, appear to aggravate the position. It has been further suggested that ulceration can develop very rapidly as a result of the excitement just prior to slaughter.

Certainly, whilst nutritional factors must not be overlooked, situations of stress must be avoided as these could, in themselves, increase acid secretion.

Minerals

The requirements vary at different stages of its life. Calcium and phosphorus are important in building up the young skeleton, and should the balance be adverse, or should there be too little of either, rickets may occur. Moreover, too high a calcium intake will tend to lock up other minerals.

A lack of manganese may cause lameness. Lack of copper and iron may cause anaemia, as we have seen. Although a copper deficiency is unlikely to occur except in unusual circumstances, this mineral is essential for normal growth and appears to improve appetite.

The pig is extremely tolerant to copper and surprisingly high levels can be fed to stock almost indefinitely. But present legislation sets a maximum inclusion level of 200 ppm per tonne and a range from 125-200 is widely adopted together with selected feed antibiotics for increasing growth rate still more. There is a considerable choice of additives for this purpose and also for the control of specific diseases such as swine dysentry, rhinitis, salmonellosis and E. coli scours.

Though rarely encountered, a deficiency of magnesium produces striking symptoms associated with weak front pasterns, sickled hocks, bowed forelegs and other symptoms resembling rickets. Hyper-irritability and muscular twitchings and a reluctance to stand have also been observed, followed by tetany and death. Growth rate is reduced as might be expected. The magnesium requirements after weaning are from 400 to 500 ppm of the total ration.

While there is some evidence to suggest that hairlessness in young pigs is due to an iodine deficiency in the sow (see also hereditary defects), a condition of goitre is sometimes encountered in older animals because this mineral is lacking. Affected pigs lose their hair and become lethargic.

To prevent this, a "rooting" mixture containing one ounce (28 g) of potassium iodide in 100 lb (45 kg) of soil can be used.

There are many proprietary mineral mixtures containing all the necessary trace elements, plus manganese, which can be incorporated in the food to avoid a deficiency and increase growth rate and there are a number of good concentrates compounded in such a way that no additional minerals need be added when the ration is balanced up with the cereal portion.

Necrotic Enteritis

From about weaning time to 16 weeks old, pigs are apt to suffer from enteritis and scouring. The condition is characterised by progressive unthriftiness, a dirty, greasy brown skin, with long hair, diarrhoea, arched back and big head. On post-mortem examination of advanced cases the large bowel is seen to be covered with an irregular, thick greyish velvety deposit which cannot be readily peeled off. Sometimes the surface shows irregular, shallow ulcers.

Owing to these characteristic changes the disease has been given the name of necrotic enteritis.

It has also been observed that a salmonella organism known as *S. suipestifer* (a member of the paratyphoid group) is sometimes present in association with these bowel changes. As a result the disease has often been called paratyphoid and the picture has become confused, for in England by far the greater number of cases of necrotic enteritis are unassociated with any paratyphoid organism.

At one time it was believed that the disease was a straightforward deficiency of nicotinic acid, and the feeding of yeast is frequently effective in some cases. Half to one cwt (25 to 50 kg) of brewers' yeast, introduced to the ton (tonne) of meal, can be used.

Some of the reported failures of yeast feeding may now be explained in the light of the recent discovery that nicotinic acid is less effective in the absence of tryptophane, one of the most important amino acids.

While the cause is not clearly understood, the affection is precipitated by cold, damp conditions towards the end of weaning and in the fattening house. If the floor is permanently wet and cold and there is too much cold air above, with indoor temperatures varying greatly during the 24 hours, then the disease is to be expected.

The malady can be prevented by avoiding such conditions, but in addition it is worth while ensuring that there is adequate vitamin A by giving an injection of 50,000 units and following up with a dose of two ounces (60 ml) of cod-liver oil. Subsequently the occurrence of the disease may be avoided by giving a weekly dose or two of pig oil. Remember necrotic enteritis is in itself not a disease but only a bowel abnormality. It is far less common today than a decade ago probably due to better housing and rations.

Greasy Pig Disease

Amongst the several skin conditions of young pigs this is the most striking when fully established. Piglets become dull and develop a 'starey' coat; then irregular, brown, soft, greasy spots develop which overlie areas of reddened skin on the snout and ears and around the eyes. These sores join up and very soon cover the whole body killing the piglet in 4-5 days. In such cases internal changes associated with the kidneys and lymph glands are often found. In milder cases recovery generally takes several weeks.

The cause is a staphylococcus commonly present in the environment, affecting some pigs in some litters but not tending to spread readily. Damage to the skin by fighting and rubbing on walls probably initiate infection.

Early treatment with injections of an antibiotic and dusting the skin with sulphanilamide powder aid recovery, but severely affected animals should be slaughtered.

Stomatic Mycosis and Gastro-enteritis

Infections associated with sores, ulcers and necrotic areas on the cheek, tongue and gums are occasionally seen in young pigs resembling analogous conditions encountered in the calf.

It is possible that a mild virus is a primary cause opening the way to infection with various bacteria including *Fusiformis necrophorus* which causes the yellowish cheesey patches characteristic of necrosis.

The condition is not serious and must not be confused with the sores which occur on the face and around the mouth thought to be associated with vitamin B deficiency, through fighting, or as a result of milk burn. External sores respond to a daily dusting with sulphonilamide powder and as the effects of the mouth changes are so slight, no treatment is justified.

The importance of fungi in foods causing mould is now well recognised (see haemorrhage scours page 97) and poisoning by aflatoxin, caused by *Aspergillus flavus*, (first recognised in turkey poults), must not be overlooked. Experimentally piglets fed contaminated food became listless, stopped eating but continued to drink and some died in 24 hours. Post-mortem showed marked liver damage. Safe levels of aflatoxin are now well recognised by food manufacturers.

Oedema
(Piglet Oedema, Gut Oedema)

Since this disease was first reported from Northern Ireland in 1951, it has been observed in widely scattered areas in England and Wales, having an irregular seasonal incidence. Initially it was encountered in piglets from eight to 14 weeks, but subsequently has been met with more and more in a much wider age group of pigs, varying from four to 20 weeks.

The symptoms are often sudden in onset, one of a group of animals being seen to throw a fit, stagger, dash its head up against a wall and vomit. The victim frequently falls on its side, pedals violently with its feet and is very soon dead. An attack is usually soon over, a small number of pigs die and the rest quickly recover. Shortly before death and in some of those that recover, the eyelids are frequently swollen and the skin of the nose puffy and soft to the touch.

POST-MORTEM FINDINGS

On post-mortem an accumulation of jelly-like material (the oedematous fluid) is to be found in various parts of the body such as the stomach wall and between the coils of the large bowel. The stomach is generally tightly packed with food. Six hours after death the fluid has drained from the gelatinous areas and is to be found freely in the body cavity—generally somewhat bloodstained.

Experimental evidence suggests that a certain serological type of beta-haemolytic *E. coli* is present in affected pigs and in in-contact pigs on infected premises, which, it is thought, under certain conditions, produce a toxin probably responsible for the symptoms. Though present in healthy pigs, it is exceedingly difficult to find as it is only there in very small numbers. It is not yet clear, however, what stimulates the initial growth of these potentially dangerous types.

Outbreaks are often associated with a marked change in feeding or management, and the disease is encountered very frequently within 10 to 14 days after pigs have been introduced to fresh premises. It is invariably the better-doing pigs of a litter or group which seem to suffer and to die first or they may do so after being introduced too quickly to a higher quality feedingstuff, and when, in addition, their movement has been restricted by adverse weather conditions or by bad management.

Oedema not uncommonly occurs when litters have been castrated, wormed and removed from their dam, all within a short space of time.

Many attempts have been made to control the disease although unfortunately few have been at all effective. Immediately a case occurs dose all surviving pigs with Epsom salts (2 oz (57 g) per 10 pigs at ten weeks of age as a guide) or give each 1 oz (30 ml) of pig oil, and deprive them of food for 24 hours, slowly bringing them back on to their full ration during the course of the next three days. The introduction of terramycin into the food sometimes helps, whether this is being fed wet or dry. Whichever it is, a change seems to be beneficial. Bearing in mind that a certain strain of *E. coli* is alleged to be responsible for the condition, some farmers have arranged for their veterinary surgeons to vaccinate all their piglets before weaning. Others have achieved success giving *E. coli* serum in anticipation of the disease or by injecting all surviving pigs with the serum three times at six-hour intervals as soon as the first pig has died. Adrenalin, anti-histamine preparations and vitamin B injections have occasionally been successful and can be given by your vet.

Your best plan to prevent oedema is to ensure that changes in feeding are made gradually. Give a weekly dose of 1 to 2 oz (30-60 ml) of pig oil during the susceptible period when pigs are adjusting themselves to their surroundings.

If you buy pigs from a market or another farm, put them on a low-quality diet at first and bring it slowly up to normal quality. And only give them half a feed when you get them on your premises, the next feed can be three-quarters of a full meal, the third and subsequent meals being full. A dose of pig oil should be given on the first day.

So far no success has been achieved in precipitating the disease by feeding a wide variety of rations. The disease is as likely to occur when pigs are being fed on potatoes and barley meal as when they are on the most highly complex and nutritious rations that can be compounded. So don't blame the food.

Salmonellosis

Much confusion has been created in the past by the use of terms such as "paratyphoid" to indicate certain conditions which did not strictly apply. Organisms of the paratyphoid group are often found in the bowel without causing any apparent harm. *S. cholerae suis* (v. Kunzendorf) has been found in association with swine fever and was regarded by some as a tracer implying that the virus of swine fever was present. This species is also found in association with necrotic enteritis, a condition for which the term "paratyphoid" has been coined. The organisms here (as with swine fever) are probably "secondary invaders", i.e. their presence is incidental but made more serious by a deterioration of the body or bowel so enabling them to establish themselves.

The number of salmonella varieties runs into dozens of which many are harmless. Some are occasionally found in raw food materials, especially those of animal origin. But when the ingredient harbouring the organism is withdrawn these organisms quickly disappear. Unfortunately more dangerous salmonellae are now appearing and causing increasing losses amongst pigs. Some stress or predisposing cause may well be present but this is not always evident. A change of buildings, variable temperature, or transportation could lower resistance. Cases tend to be prolonged rather than short-lived as the organisms are distributed about the premises, on the boots and clothing of personnel, by the movement of pigs about the premises for weighing etc, or by any movable equipment such as food barrows. While mortality may reach 15 per cent in any one week, morbidity is generally unusually high. Improvement then takes place, the condition becoming more chronic, but many pigs remain carriers of the organism, harbouring it in their intestinal glands. *S. typhimurium* and *S. dublin* are particularly involved in such cases, the former being the more pathogenic.

SYMPTOMS

These occur usually in 60-100 lb (27-45 kg) pigs and include inappetence with recumbency, some animals showing a high temperature with typical nettle-rash appearance of the skin. There is constipation rather than scouring, particularly with those showing high temperatures. Skin changes consisting of raised patches of purple scabs scattered along the sides and flanks are frequently seen. In other cases there may be diffuse blue-to-purple discoloration of the ears, feet and parts of the skin. This form is usually fatal and has been described previously as "blue pig disease". *S. dublin* may also cause meningitis.

Apart from the absence of scouring many features of salmonellosis (especially the post-mortem changes) resemble swine fever. But with the virtual elimination of the latter disease confusion can no longer occur and a greater awareness of the existence of salmonellosis will ensure a more rapid diagnosis.

TREATMENT

The importance of a proper diagnosis based on a post-mortem and bacteriological test cannot be over-emphasised, and at any time a bacteriological examination of faeces will help to establish the type of bacterium and its sensitivity to available drugs. Some of the newer antibiotics such as ampicillin are proving effective.

Bought-in animals should be confined on arrival for 2-3 weeks and all groups on the farm isolated as far as possible, movement being restricted to a minimum. Any system such as sowstalls, individual feeders, birth-to-slaughter pens, is an advantage in this respect, reducing the chances of spread of infection. The disinfection and resting of the premises after use must receive careful attention. Fortunately, however, there is now an excellent vaccine (Suscovax) which when used in combination with good management and hygiene can reduce losses to an absolute minimum.

Risks of Swill Feeding

As the feeding of swill to pigs is a practice which is likely to continue, it is important that the risks associated with this system should be understood.

In the first place there is a legal obligation to boil all swill* and maintain it at boiling temperature for at least one hour in order to destroy infective material. It may contain the viruses of swine fever, foot-and-mouth disease, swine vesicular disease, fowl pest and salmonella bacteria.

And remember that household scraps, hotel waste, etc, should be similarly treated. Further, don't put boiled swill into unsterilised containers or mix it with raw swill. Processed swill is now widely used and is prepared under licence.

While it is desirable that the person who mixes and boils the swill should have no direct contact with the animals, this is often impossible; but at least the person concerned can put on clean rubber boots and clean overalls and wash his hands thoroughly before attending to feeding.

Nutritional disorders arising from swill feeding also have to be considered.

The composition of swill varies greatly, even from the same source. It may at one time contain much bread, at another a high proportion of cabbage and greenstuff, and on another occasion meat or fish scraps and offal. Sometimes there is a

* *Disease of Animals Acts (Boiling of Animal Foodstuffs) Order of 1977.*

high fat content. This should be skimmed from the top after the swill is cooled and before feeding it to the pigs. If fed, it will reduce appetite and lower the efficiency of food conversion and may lead to an "oily" carcase.

Owing to its high fibre content, swill should be introduced gradually and not before the pigs reach 12 weeks of age. Further, as it is usually low in protein, up to 10 per cent fish or meat meal should be incorporated in the meal balancer. But check the quality of the swill first before supplementing it or you may unbalance it still further.

Swill is generally low in minerals and is likely to have little vitamin A or D; therefore the addition of a little cod-liver oil, one fluid oz (28 ml) per pig, added direct to the trough once weekly until the pigs are 140 lb (63 kg) liveweight, is desirable. Powdered and stabilised vitamin supplements are also available. An ounce or two (28-57 g) of yeast per animal will bolster up the protein and one or two per cent of a mixed mineral supplement in the food is probably the best way of adjusting the latter. To ensure that none of these "bits and pieces" are lacking you should balance up with one of the best animal protein "concentrates" now on the market.

One risk of swill feeding is salt poisoning. See chapter 11 for tackling this trouble.

Chapter 7

DISEASES DUE TO PARASITES

THERE are two types of parasitic infections—internal and external—in the pig. Internal ones are due to lung worms, stomach worms and bowel worms; external infections are caused by lice and mange.

Round Worms

Up until about 1965 the worms most commonly found in pigs were the round worms scientifically known as ascarids—*Ascaris suis*. These may be as much as 12 in (300 mm) long and nearly ¼ in (6 mm) thick. They are generally to be found in the small bowel, but some may penetrate into the stomach and occasionally up into the liver via the bile duct.

The female worm lays as many as 200,000 eggs per day, which pass out in the droppings. Under ideal, warm, damp conditions these become infective in eight weeks, but in adverse conditions this may take many months.

Infection is contracted by eating material contaminated with the embryonated eggs. These hatch in the bowel and the liberated larvae make their way via the liver to the lungs. A few may pass via the placenta into the uterus, so that in exceptional circumstances infection may occur in this way before birth.

Their passage through the lungs causes small haemorrhages

Subsequently the larvae are coughed up and swallowed, ultimately reaching the bowel once more, where they stay and grow to maturity.

Worm infection causes trouble in young pigs between three and four months of age. Coughing usually occurs; this is often severe and the chest movements so exaggerated that such piglets are known to farmers as "pankers". Some say they have got "the thumps" (see also anaemia). In the most severe cases death may follow in a few days, but usually animals fail to grow and remain unthrifty and stunted.

Other symptoms are diarrhoea, straining—even eversion of the rectum—and colic. Affected pigs are usually pot-bellied.

Secondary organisms may set up bronchial catarrh, snuffles and possibly pneumonia, but the latter is rarely a consequence of round worm invasion.

On post-mortem examination haemorrhagic spots may be seen in the lungs, indicating recent invasion and in older pigs (at least several weeks after invasion) the liver frequently shows what are known as "milk spots". These are diffuse white areas, up to the size of 1p piece, which have been caused by the passage of the larvae when migrating. The minute network of liver lobules can be seen outlined in white.

Occasionally immature parasites may dam back the bile, in the bile duct, which results in jaundice with a yellowing of the skin and the mucous membranes.

The disease has become so serious in some parts of the USA that the Federal Bureau of Animal Industry in co-operation with farmers has devised a system of sanitation which farmers are asked to follow.

GETTING RID OF ROUND WORMS

The system is:

1. Clean the farrowing pen thoroughly with hot soda water (2lb (900 g) of washing soda to 30 gallons (136 litres) of boiling water) in preparation for the sow. It should be allowed to dry out, of course, before adding bedding.

2. Before bringing her in to farrow, add worm remedy to food

and 24 hours later scrub her thoroughly with soapy water to remove all dirt from her body and udder.

3. Put the sow in the clean pen. Do not allow her to walk over infected ground in between.

4. If outdoor system, place clean houses or huts on clean ground.

5. Haul the sow and pigs to clean ground. Do not drive them over the old paddocks.

You will note that I have given most of the recommended steps in chapter 3 as part of the normal before-farrowing management.

Now other bowel parasites have replaced *A.suis* in importance and remedies have become more effective; when added to the food these remove all the bowel and stomach parasites both adult and immature. These drugs are safe and effective if used properly. But good hygienic measures will go a long way to reducing infestation to a low level.

An egg-laying pattern has now been discovered which is common to all this group. There is a rapid rise in numbers, particularly of *O. dentatum* eggs, commencing just before farrowing, this being maintained but tailing off as suckling proceeds and ultimately ceasing. The rise and fall is more closely related to suckling than to any other factor. The egg count bears no close relationship to the number of worms present, but is a useful general guide to the degree of infestation.

Worm infestation is essentially a herd problem but can only be solved if premises are properly disinfected before clean stock are introduced and the correct treatment is applied at the right time. Animals kept largely on concrete are just as likely to harbour infection if hygiene is not scrupulous, as animals on pasture.

Treatment of the sow should take place as mentioned just before farrowing and piglets likewise at 7-12 weeks of age.

PIG-SICK PASTURES

After a variable time, which may be anything from 18 months to two years according to the rate of stocking and type and extent of disease present, pastures become what is known as "pig sick". Whilst it is accepted that this is mainly due to increasing contamination with the eggs of worms, other diseases may well play a part. In practice the beneficial effect of a change-over to new pasture has often been reported even if no specific disease condition has existed. It is thus most important to adopt some system of rotation. To rest the buildings occasionally is also an advantage (see under scouring).

As far as *Ascaris suis* is concerned the eggs are particularly resistant to climatic conditions and take many months to die. So do ensure that a pig pasture comes under the plough every three or four years and is cropped for a year or two before being laid down again to grass for further pig grazing. In general, it is inadvisable to graze pigs on a pasture for more than two years running, even if some system of rotation has been adopted.

Indoor premises can, as I have explained, be readily cleansed by thorough scraping and washing and by the subsequent application of hot soda solution (two oz (60 g) of washing soda in two gallons (9 litres) of water).

Lung Worms

Pigs sometimes suffer from the presence of worms in the lung tubes. These are white and very slender, look like threads of white cotton and may be two inches to three inches (50 to 75 mm) long. They cause considerable irritation and coughing, which may lead to pneumonia. The infection seems to occur mostly with pigs kept in dark, damp conditions that have access to a pig-sick paddock.

The female worm lays her eggs in the lungs. These are coughed up and swallowed, and by the time they have reached the outside world in droppings they are already hatched. They are then eaten by earthworms where they undergo two changes before they become infective.

One earthworm may harbour as many as 2,000 larvae and when eaten can be responsible for a heavy infection in the pig. After passing from the bowel the larvae reach the lungs once again.

Pigs that appear sound and healthy can carry these worms, and these may only cause trouble if the animal becomes sick

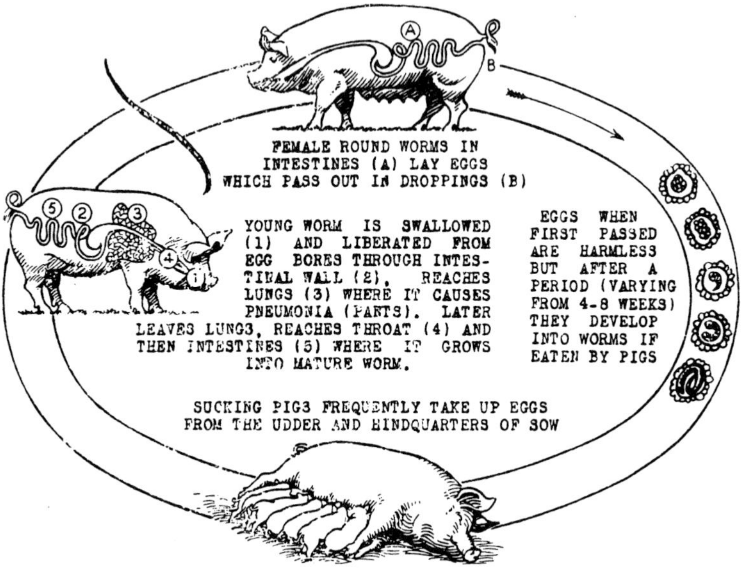

THE COMMON PIG WORM

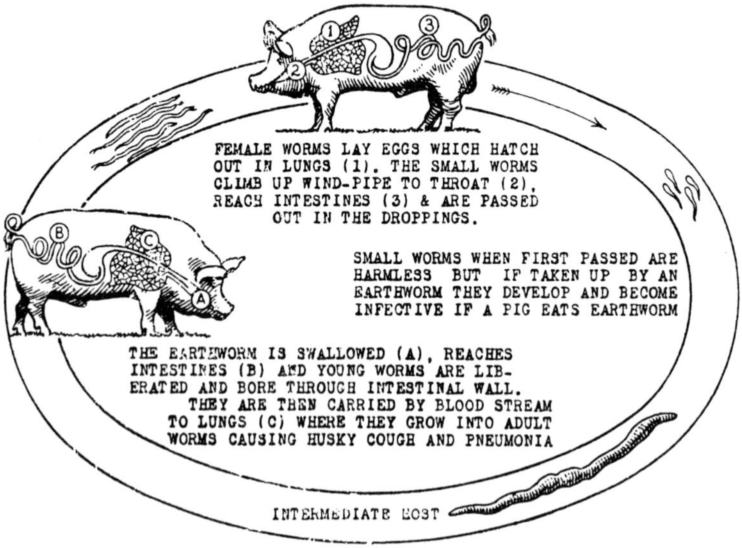

LUNG WORM OF THE PIG

from some other cause. Less strong pigs may go down more quickly, especially if the infestation is heavy.

The symptoms are generally those of coughing, the pigs becoming thin and weak. They develop a rough coat and are unthrifty.

Control largely depends on sanitary measures and a rotation of pastures. But pigs can also be drenched with Helmox, a preparation containing inactivated irradiated larvae. Some idea of the degree of infection of a pasture can be obtained by collecting several earthworms and having them examined for their larval content at a laboratory.

Tape Worm (*Cysticercus cellulosae*)

While tape worm infection of pigs is extremely rare, the bladder stage or cyst of a tape worm is to be found in the muscles of the tongue and other parts of the body.

Human beings contract the infection, especially in the USA and many European countries where pig flesh is eaten lightly cooked. The tape worm *T. solium* develops from the cysts. Pigs pick up the eggs when exposed to material contamination by human excreta.

Since the establishment of prisoner-of-war and refugee camps in this country following the war the incidence of *Cysticercosis* has increased, but so long as our meat is properly cooked tape-worm infestation in the human population will remain at a low level. However, the hazard of such infection is now greater than it used to be.

Stomach and Intestinal Worms

There is only one stomach worm to be found affecting pigs in Great Britain (*Hyostrongylus rubidus*). Infection is increasingly common. When it does occur it may give rise to marked inflammation and a lowering of general condition.

The worm is a small, red thread-like creature, less than half an inch (12 mm) in length but readily seen against the stomach wall.

The life history is direct, it being possible for animals to re-infect themselves.

This parasite, *O. dentatum*, and *T. suis* are thought to be associated with "the thin sow syndrome".

Suckling sows quite often become emaciated and start scouring as result of an infection with "rubidum". A very effective remedy for strongyloid worms is Thibenzole, but there are now several good remedies on the market to choose from.

Whip Worm (*Trichuris suis*)

This worm is attached by a long slender thread, rather like a whip, to the mucous membrane of the blind gut or caecum, and large bowel. Here the adult lays its eggs. These pass out in the dung where they develop. Under ideal conditions of warmth and moisture, mature infective larvae may be developed in three weeks. When eaten these find their way to the lower bowel where they attach themselves to the gut wall.

A heavy infestation of this parasite can be responsible for and associated with clinical symptoms of emaciation and scouring. Its habit of attaching itself deeply to the gut lining is thought to enable bacteria such as *E. coli*, salmonella and various "vibrios" to establish themselves and to create symptoms such as are characteristic of swine dysentery. In other words, the presence of large numbers of *T. suis* may be the trigger mechanism for several forms of enteric disease and explain the erratic nature of their appearance. The parasite can also be responsible, on its own account, for severe emaciation in pigs, especially following weaning.

Nodular Worm (*Oesophagostomum dentatum*)

This worm, to be found in the small bowel, is becoming more common and may be found in large numbers. It may, however, in conjunction with other parasites, cause inflammation and interfere with digestion. It is 1-1½ in (25-37 mm) long.

The larva burrows into the mucous membrane and produces small nodules. In 40 days it becomes mature and returns into the bowel. If the infection is heavy it may be responsible for a condition known as "pimply gut". Such small pimples can develop into small abscesses and may cause trouble. The piperazine preparations are not effective in controlling these parasites.

The above three thread worms may be responsible for vomiting, emaciation, scouring and irregular heats or complete cessation of heat periods. An examination of the dung will reveal the extent of the infection as reflected in the total egg count.

Modern worm remedies are very effective. *Ascaris suis* and the lungworm can be removed by an injection, and the remaining bowel worms by adding the remedy to the food. For advice as to what to use, check with your veterinary surgeon.

Trichinosis

This trouble is very rarely met with in this country though sporadic outbreaks may occur and some cases probably go undetected.

The worm involved (*Trichinella spiralis*) spends its short existence of about six weeks in the small bowel of pigs. Eggs are laid in the lining where they hatch and migrate to the muscles, here becoming encysted. Pig flesh eaten raw can cause infection in humans and very severe rheumatic pains in the muscles. The main source of infection of pigs is rats which keep the disease going among themselves by cannibalism.

Coccidiosis

The condition is by no means so rare in Great Britain as was originally believed. Possibly the similarity between it and swine dysentery has helped to conceal its existence. It is commonly encountered in pigs of from 12 to 16 weeks of age. The parasite responsible (*Isospora suis*) attacks the bowel wall causing shedding of the surface mucous membrane. This material may accumulate in the bowel so that the wall becomes thick and the bowel like a piece of stiff rubber piping.

There is first diarrhoea followed by constipation, then loss of appetite and progressive unthriftiness. In more chronic cases, the dung may be dark brown and flecked with blood. Treatment with sulphamezathine, either in the form of pills or by injection, is very effective, bringing about a cure in 24 to 48 hours. The amount given depends upon the weight of the pig and the concentration of the solution respectively. Where premises are contaminated by infected pigs, disinfection with household ammonia is satisfactory. The oocysts are quickly destroyed by a 10 per cent solution. As in other domestic animals and in birds, the coccidium of the pig is specific and does not affect any other species. Neither can the pig contract infection from infected birds or animals.

Leptospirosis (*L. icterohaemorrhagiae*)

The existence of this disease has only been recognised in recent times. It is due to a microscopic parasite resembling a tiny piece of twisted wire. Rats are the normal carriers of this parasite, which they liberate in their urine. There is always the risk of infection on rat-infested premises.

The condition may be sub-clinical in the sow, resulting later in abortion. Alternatively, many piglets may be born weak or die a few days or weeks after birth. The sow may have a temperature of 104°F (40°C).

When the parasites invade the body, the liver and the kidneys are particularly affected and jaundice may occur. Later, infection tends to localise in the kidneys, and large numbers of parasites are passed out in the pig's urine. Occasionally dogs and humans become infected and the former may transmit the disease to pigs.

The death rate is generally low but affected pigs look very sick, lose their appetite and are often described as suffering from "the yellows". Streptomycin is a most effective remedy. It can be injected in the first instance and repeated in several days' time.

Whilst in pigs in England *L. icterohaemorrhagiae* is the organism which causes the trouble, the pig is known to be a carrier of *L. pomona* in New Zealand, conveying infection to calves. The pig itself is seldom affected. Reports from South Africa indicate that another species, *S. suilla*, is responsible for a rather acute type of spirochaetosis in pigs in that country, gaining access to the body through wounds, particularly those associated with castration and cutting of the teeth. It results in a characteristic swelling of the sides of the nostrils and lower jaw, with abscess formation in the nasal passages. *S. suilla* seems to be very much more pathogenic than its counterpart in England and more ubiquitous. It can also produce swellings under the skin which may ulcerate and do not heal readily on their own.

Toxoplasma (*T. gondii*)

T. gondii has only recently been recorded as a cause of wasting and respiratory distress in piglets. The parasite is to be found causing damage to the lungs, liver, kidneys and lymph nodes.

Whilst young piglets of only a few weeks of age appear to be most susceptible and suffer from the acute respiratory form, adults may also be affected and be observed shivering and coughing and showing signs of incoordination of movement, relaxation of the abdominal muscles and diarrhoea. Such animals become listless and may succumb to the infection. The source of this parasite has yet to be determined.

Chapter 8

SKIN AFFECTIONS

Lice

LARGE black lice, readily visible to the naked eye, are quite frequently seen on the skin of pigs. These are not known to do any harm and are to be found even on thriving animals. If present in large numbers they may, however, cause unrest and unthriftiness and they can carry the virus of pig pox.

Barley straw, although commonly accused of causing a rash, cannot be blamed as a source of the trouble. Where it appears to be associated with marked skin irritation, especially in the summer-time, the possibility of heavy contamination with harvest mites must not be overlooked attached singly to the hairs.

The odd pig or two may be dressed with old sump oil or pig oil, but where a large number of animals are involved it is far simpler and more effective to use one of the modern insecticides containing benzine hexachloride which can be made up in a watery solution and sprayed on by a stirrup-pump. As the pig has no thick coat, the effects are limited to a few weeks. Spraying should therefore be repeated in about 3 weeks in order to destroy the next generation emerging from the eggs which were present during the initial treatment.

Where pigs are infected, the premises are also likely to be contaminated, so that it is a good plan also to spray the pen.

About an hour after spraying the pigs, remove them to clean premises, then collect together and burn the litter they left behind; spray the pen with the same solution as used for the pigs and allow to dry out before putting in fresh bedding and stock.

Mange

Sarcoptic mange, such as is encountered in dogs and horses, is commonly met with in pigs of all ages. Infestation may be severe or mild in both young and old pigs. With young pigs it may be so severe as completely to prevent normal rest. The entire skin surface may be grey and sticky. In older animals the condition may produce a widespread reddening and pimply formation of the skin, causing them to rub persistently against the sides of their pen.

The parasite is just visible to the naked eye when crawling on a black surface. It burrows under the skin, causing small irritant papules, which encourage the pig to rub. Sore areas may be produced. The skin becomes rough and wrinkled and the animal may become unthrifty and weak. Diagnosis can readily be established by examining several skin scrapings from affected parts. When the material is put in a caustic soda solution and boiled, the hair and extraneous matter is dissolved and the parasites can be seen in the residue when examined under a microscope.

If the scabs are few, wash the parts with soap and water and apply an ointment containing benzyl benzoate. If one of the readily available preparations containing BHC is employed, improvement will occur. As in the treatment of lice, a liquid preparation is preferable. The entire animal should be sprayed, special attention being paid to the ears which should be swabbed with cotton wool soaked in the solution, as here is the usual reservoir of infection—particularly in sows and boars.

Where mange is persistent it is worth immersing each piglet at weaning time for three seconds in a bath of anti-mange solution, holding it by the hind legs.

Specific Skin Rash (Parakeratosis)

Although this condition is not associated with any known

parasite, it is included here because in the early stage it can be so readily confused with mange, and it is most difficult to make a correct differential diagnosis.

This type of dermatitis (also known as dirty-skin disease) occurs in pigs which have been brought into the fattening house about a fortnight and from 12 to 16 weeks of age. It tends to spread along the back and down the hind legs, being especially marked around the region of the hock, both front and back. Dust and food material tend to stick to the natural grease of the skin and accumulate until a thick, scurfy area, often described as "elephant skin" has developed. At this stage the general appearance of the pig has become unthrifty, the hair long and the skin dark. There may be some scouring. Obviously the general health of the animal is affected and usually such animals take from three to four weeks longer to reach bacon weight.

This type of skin rash, strangely enough, is closely related to *ad lib* dry feeding and it is difficult to explain why it tends to disappear within a few weeks when feeding is restricted, or where wet feeding is introduced.

Since American work indicated the relationship between zinc and non-specific skin rashes, abundant evidence has accumulated to confirm this finding. Whilst ordinary, non-supplemented foods may contain from 30 to 40 parts per million of zinc, under certain conditions, especially those of *ad lib* dry feeding, this amount appears to be insufficient—or possibly unavailable to the pig. The situation can, however, be remedied, with advantage, by adding zinc in the form of zinc carbonate (about ½ lb (227 g) per ton) so that the level is increased to 150 to 200 parts per million. Even with this amount present it would seem that a high calcium content can interfere with absorption, thus causing the rash to appear.

Ringworm (*Microsporum nanum*)

Infection of pigs with the ringworm fungus is relatively rare. Pigs that are affected show marked raised grey, sticky areas, roughly circular in shape with a reddish margin. On other occasions the ringworm plaques may be more irregular and take the form of wavy reddish eczematous lines or patches which may cover large areas of the body.

Whilst the condition is resistant to treatment, showing but poor response to the application of fungicides or iodine, it does not spread very readily from animal to animal.

Griseofulvin is now being used successfully in the form of an injection or as an ointment, for the control of ringworm. After animals have been treated and recovered, their pens should be thoroughly soaked in hot soda solution, allowed to dry and sprayed over with a fungicide before fresh stock is introduced.

Pityriasis Rosea

This condition is characterised in its latter stages by a striking "marbled" appearance of the belly and underparts of the pig. Animals from 6-12 weeks are most frequently affected, but quite commonly only one or two in a batch appear to suffer.

The first indication of its presence is the appearance of small pin-point crusts distributed widely over the affected area. These extend and develop in a horseshoe manner similar to classical ringworm in the human, until ridges in the shape of circles or part circles are formed over the affected area. The crusts then decay, leaving a mosaic-like pattern, which looks as though it has been traced with a hot poker point.

This condition, still quite rare in the United Kingdom, has been known for some time in Norway where it is considered to be an hereditary disease. Every effort to transmit it has failed, affected animals recovering spontaneously. It is of little or no economic importance as bodily growth is unaffected.

Papular Dermatitis

This condition, whose name is a description of the condition, must not be confused with mange or the early stages of parakeratosis. It is due to a fungus of the aspergillus group and is associated with contaminated litter and poor hygiene.

Dermatosis Vegetans

The first cases of this disease were seen in Britain in 1958 and a few cases have been encountered since.

Pigs of from 3 to 8 weeks old are chiefly affected. There are marked changes seen on the skin, abnormalities of the feet, and respiratory disturbances. The skin changes are commonly seen at two to three weeks of age but may occasionally be noticed at birth. They start as raised, pink circumscribed areas, usually on the abdomen or inside the thighs, but occasionally on the back and sides. They develop through a stage resembling *Pityriasis rosea*, coalesce and are covered with a yellowish-brown, brittle material. The skin becomes thick and cracks appear in the crusts. The changes slowly disappear but can persist for many months. There is no irritation and local treatment of sores only is justified as these are likely to become infected.

The appearance of the feet resembles club-foot, being markedly swollen and the skin rotted and thickened well above the hoof edge.

The condition is usually fatal in 4 to 6 weeks after the onset, there being marked respiratory disturbance in the latter stages.

Non-Specific Skin Rash (Pseudo-Parakeratosis)

This condition occasionally encountered in adolescent and fully grown animals appears to be associated with a low energy diet where there is a shortage of essential fatty acids, in particular linoleic acid.

Cases are usually associated with marked environmental stress such as arises in draughty buildings with cold damp floors and no bedding. This may be part of the thin sow syndrome but there is here, in addition, marked loss of hair revealing a bare cracked skin with irregular sores, especially along the back. Brownish secretions accumulate in the axillae and behind the ears. The distribution and nature of the skin changes distinguish this condition from classical parakeratosis and response to linoleic acid is good.

Greasy Pig Disease

(See page 101.)

Chapter 9

SOME RESPIRATORY, VIRUS AND BACTERIAL INFECTIONS

I PROPOSE to begin this chapter by dealing with the respiratory diseases of the pig. The first thing to emphasise is the difficulty of accurate diagnosis.

Coughing is a symptom of respiratory disease; but it is also associated with other conditions. Indeed, it is a common symptom of about five complaints:

1. It is characteristic (to a certain extent) of fattening houses and although careful experiments have shown that it is not easy to establish chronic coughing by exposing piglets to air heavily laden with dust particles, there is usually a certain amount of meal blown about and odd pigs are apt to show signs of temporary irritation. In contrast to this, the absence of coughing in conditions of high humidity, as in the "sweat-box" system, is remarkable.

2. In the young animal it is common in pneumonia resulting from swine fever, rhinitis, enzootic pneumonia and toxo-plasmosis.

3. It is characteristic of worm infestation and is associated with the stage during which the worm larvae pass through the lungs.

4. Pneumonia associated with pasteurella organisms.

5. In pigs of 100 lb (45 kg) and over it is mainly associated with enzootic pneumonia, although there appear to

be other non-specific forms which cause a similar disturbance.

Therefore, in cases of coughing where there are no other symptoms to aid the diagnosis, it is necessary first to consider the possibility of worm infestation or the more simple matter of dust-laden air being responsible or to decide whether the condition is a follow-on from swine fever (which is dealt with in a later chapter) and to study the environmental conditions. In this respect a study of the "sweat-box" system in which there is no draught, and in which the atmosphere is relatively stagnant (79-80°F/26°C) and the air 100 per cent saturated with moisture vapour, deserves serious consideration. Undoubtedly such conditions are comfortable to the pig, for coughing is the exception. Under such conditions it is thought that bacteria and virus particles become swollen, and are more readily carried down by the water of condensation in which the obnoxious ammonia is also presumably dissolved.

Enzootic Pneumonia

Undoubtedly there are a number of conditions covered by the old name VPP which vary only slightly in practice on the farm but which are histologically distinct. The cause of enzootic pneumonia is now known to be a mycoplasma (*M. hyopneumoniae*) and not a virus. The incubation period is 10-15 days.

The condition is found in its most prominent form in fattening pigs from three months onwards. It can, however, affect pigs right from birth. The symptoms in early life may be overlooked as they are usually very mild. It is widespread throughout the country, some 60 per cent of pig farms still being affected—this figure being even higher in some areas. The disease spreads from pig to pig mainly by direct contact and does not seem to spread in any other way. Under dry conditions fine particles are formed and penetrate deep into the lungs. Under warm, humid conditions the droplets are larger and less likely to get beyond the upper respiratory tract. In the suckling pig symptoms may be very mild indeed, but after four or five weeks of age, lachrymation and sneezing, with occasional coughing on being disturbed, may be all that there is to indicate the presence of the disease. While the disease is not fatal at this stage, pigs may be unthrifty.

In pigs from 14 weeks onwards, the disease generally assumes the chronic form, symptoms rapidly subside, but there is quite often a re-appearance around about 20 weeks. Recovered pigs subsequently remain carriers for a year or more. Deaths are rare, but as a rule pigs become unthrifty—and unprofitable. The retardation of growth rate has been reported to be 14–16 per cent, and food conversion rate is adversely affected.

At slaughter, characteristic dark-red solid areas depressed below the surrounding lung tissue can be seen. These are firm to the touch, limited in size and often widely dispersed. The small, front pendulous lobes are frequently affected.

CONTROL MEASURES

Undoubtedly good feeding and management reduce the ravages of this disease to a minimum. This is borne out by the observation that many farmers are unaware from their records of rate of growth and grading that the disease is present.

It is possible, by rigorous isolation of each breeding animal and by keeping the litters separate to bacon weight, to identify the carrier animals, which as a rule show no symptoms, and so eradicate the disease. The lungs of the offspring are examined.

Farrowing and rearing in isolation would be ideal, but such strict supervision very often necessitates additional labour and the plan is not always practicable.

Experiments have, however, shown that infection does not persist for more than a day or two in pens recently occupied by infected animals. If left untouched for 48 hours, the agent will die of its own accord, but it is better to make quite certain before putting fresh pigs into such a pen to clean it out (after it has been shut up for 48 hours) and then to spray the walls and floor with hot washing soda (1 handful to 1 gallon (4·5 l) of boiling water), allow to dry out, then swill out with clean fresh water and allow to dry out once more before again re-stocking.

It is often difficult to identify the disease in litters running with affected sows. If the former are chased vigorously, some may be persuaded to cough before the pursuer is exhausted! In general it is better to run each litter as a unit through to bacon weight, overlooking for the time being what is clearly a sound practical point, namely, mixing pigs from different litters in uniform batches.

If you want to clear the disease you must take some trouble, so keep the litters separate and have them inspected by a veterinary surgeon at slaughter. Then you would be able to check back on each sow or gilt and decide which should be disposed of and which should be kept. One piglet may be sacrificed at weaning. If there is any disease present, the use of Tylan for a week before the change and a week after, as an anti-stress remedy, is to be recommended.

To reduce the spread of infection in the piggery, the pen walls should be built up to at least 5 ft (1·5 m) or preferably to the ceiling, but whatever you do, ensure satisfactory ventilation. Reducing ventilation rate can easily exacerbate the condition. Cold damp conditions encourage the spread and survival of the disease. Food fed wet and warm helps to ease coughing spasms.

In view of the widespread nature of the disease, farmers who have at present a clean herd should avoid buying in stock which are obviously affected by some respiratory trouble and make inquiries beforehand as to the health of the herd. It is possible for boars to become infected when mating, but this risk can be largely avoided by using a service crate.

Through the enterprise of a number of pig farmers an organisation known as the Pig Health Control Association provides an opportunity for those who wish to avail themselves of all existing knowledge regarding the disease, methods of eradication, and ways of building up an enzootic pneumonia free herd.

There is an increasing number of clean herds which provide a valuable source of supply for those wishing to start clean herds from scratch, and the establishment of several herds from MD stock is already having a marked impact on the industry. Clean animals on to new premises is the ideal way to start. On the other hand, running a herd where all sow have had three or four litters can much improve matters as immunity develops with age. Future stock is best selected from these sows rather than from gilts.

X1 Disease

The successful eradication of enzootic pneumonia from many herds has revealed, in a small number of cases, the presence of a respiratory disease not hitherto generally recognised in the United Kingdom. It is undoubtedly widespread but sparse in distribution.

The condition is a form of rhinitis, affecting both young and old pigs, associated with generalised sneezing and slight unthriftiness. Organisms such as *Bordetella bronchisepticus and Haemophylus suis*, associated generally with chronic infections, are usually to be found. Antibiotic therapy is beneficial.

Hysterectomy

The vast majority of pigs are born into the world free of the common diseases, but quickly become "contaminated" when exposed to their normal environment. If, however, they can be removed from the uterus of their dam directly into a sterilised environment and under rigorously controlled conditions, there is a good guarantee of their remaining free, for at least a period during which they are kept strictly isolated, from enzootic pneumonia, rhinitis, parasitic mange and certain forms of non-specific bacterial infection which are known to constitute a serious hazard to pigs born naturally on the farm.

The method already extensively used in the United States is as follows:

The selected sow is removed to the operating theatre approximately two days before anticipated farrowing. She is anaesthetised by exposure to liquid carbon dioxide; the belly, previously disinfected, is opened and the entire uterus removed aseptically after being tightly tied at the stalk. The contained mass of foetuses is dropped into a disinfectant bath and slipped under a vane into a sterilised chamber, where operators remove the piglets one by one and put them in polythene bags. These are then removed to the other end and conveyed to appropriate cages where the piglets are reared from two to six weeks on sterile food in sterile containers.

Piglets reared in this fashion appear to grow equally well if not better than naturally-born animals. When exposed to the natural hazards on a reasonably good farm they do not seem to suffer from lack of early exposure which may be considered to have given them early immunity or resistance to certain infections.

In order that such a process should give maximum results it should undoubtedly be carried out by competent authorities, employing experienced veterinary surgeons, and pigs should only be issued, at least in the early stages of this venture, to those farmers who have had no pigs on their premises for six months, or who are starting new ventures.

In the latter class can be included the central breeding stations owned by a "group", taking first-generation minimal-disease pigs and supplying their members with in-pig gilts.

In such cases every reasonable precaution should be taken to prevent the introduction of disease. Visiting parties are strictly taboo. The fewer people who enter the premises the better, and all who do—the veterinary surgeon not excepted—should pass through a decontamination chamber. No member of the staff should keep pigs, and there should be no pig farmers in the vicinity bordering the perimeter. All materials should be off-loaded outside the entrance to the establishment from a vehicle which has passed through a disinfectant bath.

Hysterectomy has, however, not achieved the popularity originally anticipated for a number of reasons. The cost of production has been higher than expected because of the high proportion of piglets failing to grow adequately after birth. Weakness and retarded growth suggest some deficiency or obscure infection. Furthermore, the conditions which such piglets need to develop their maximum potential are not at all easy to secure and maintain, and finally health standards throughout the industry have, in general, greatly improved so that it is possible to secure stock at common market prices

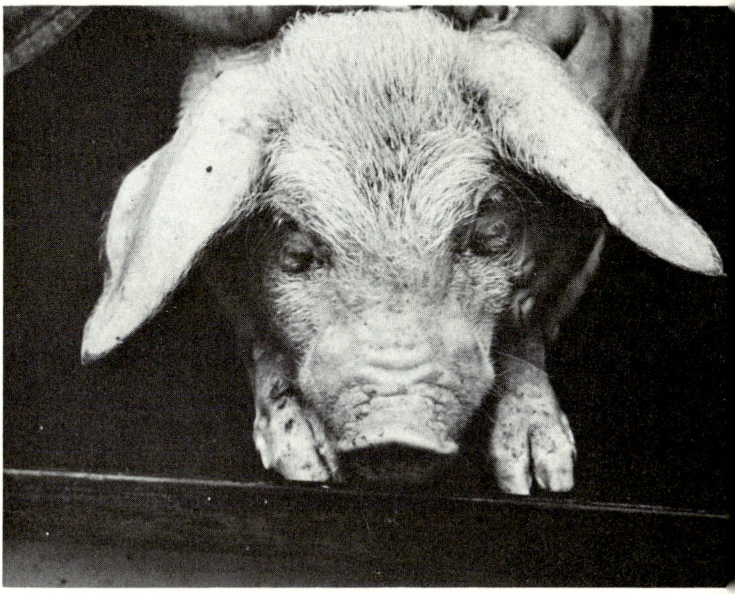

Atrophic rhinitis in a young piglet. Externally the snout appears swollen and twisted. X-ray examination revealed total atrophy of the bone on both sides of the snout.

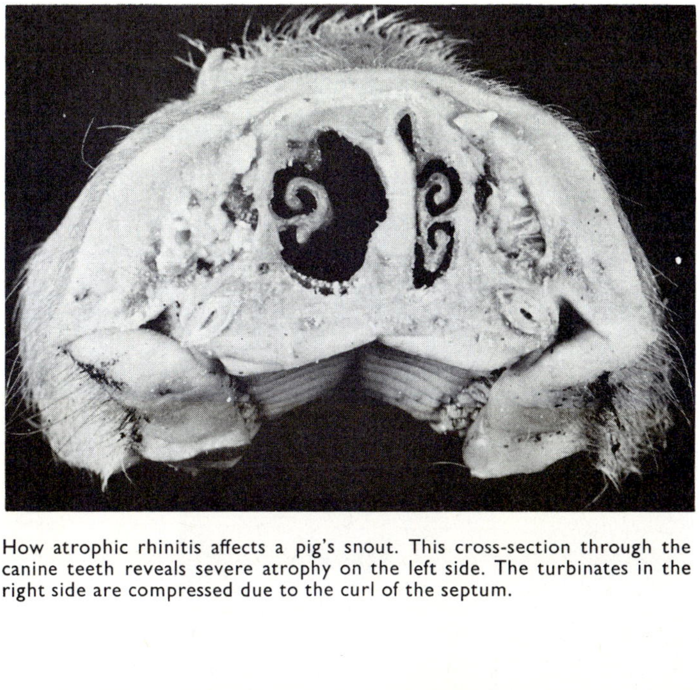

How atrophic rhinitis affects a pig's snout. This cross-section through the canine teeth reveals severe atrophy on the left side. The turbinates in the right side are compressed due to the curl of the septum.

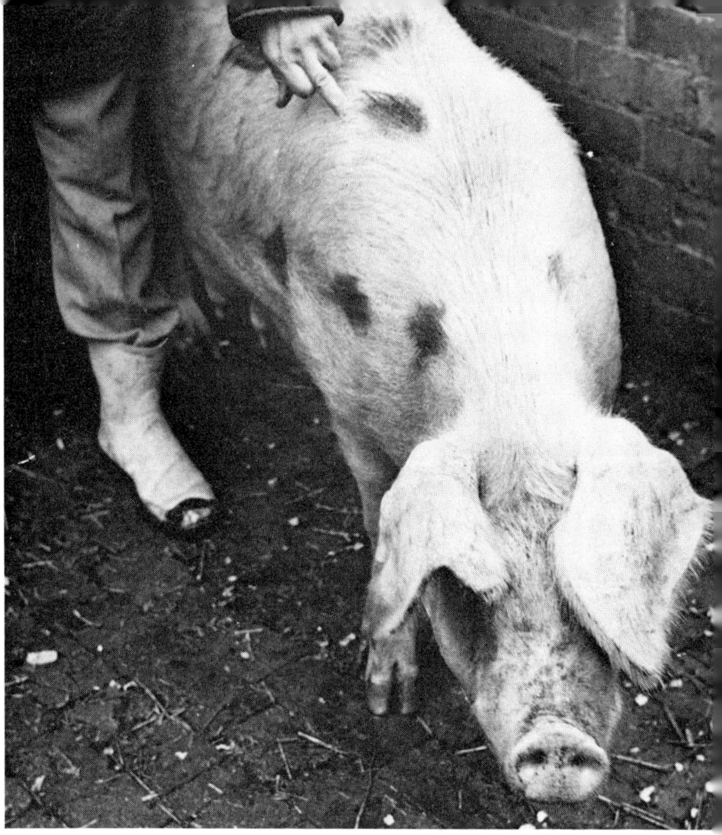

Characteristic diamond markings or plaques on the skin of a pig suffering from the sub-acute form of erysipelas. Most pigs affected with this form of the disease recover.

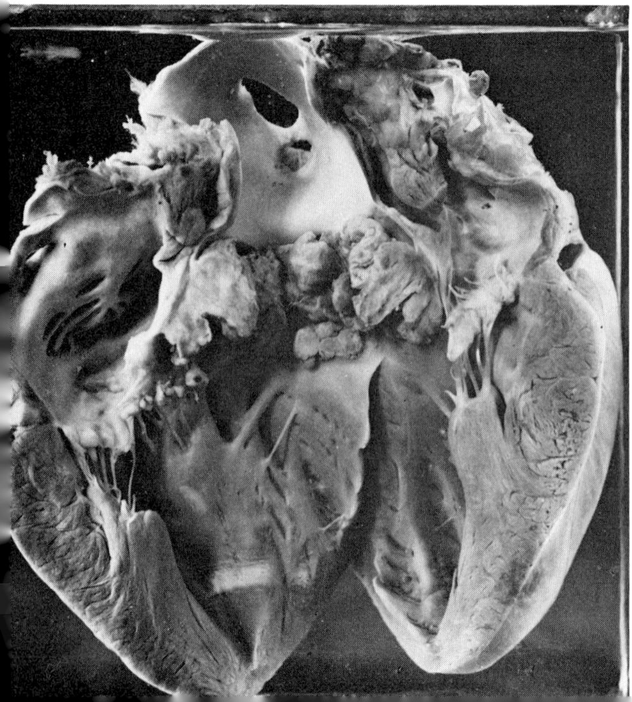

Erysipelas infection of the heart. Note cauliflower-like growth on valves separating upper and lower chambers of the heart.

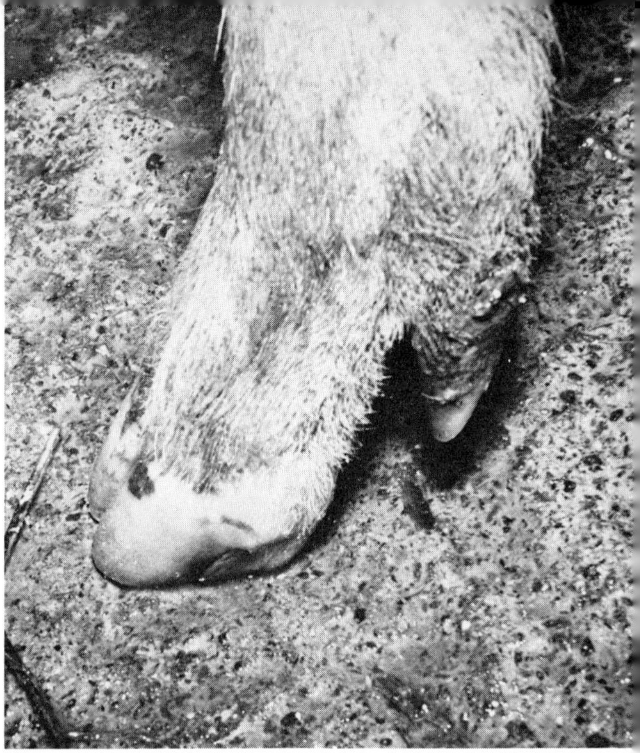

Concrete floors that are too rough can wear away the foot and cause a false sand-crack, and consequent lameness.

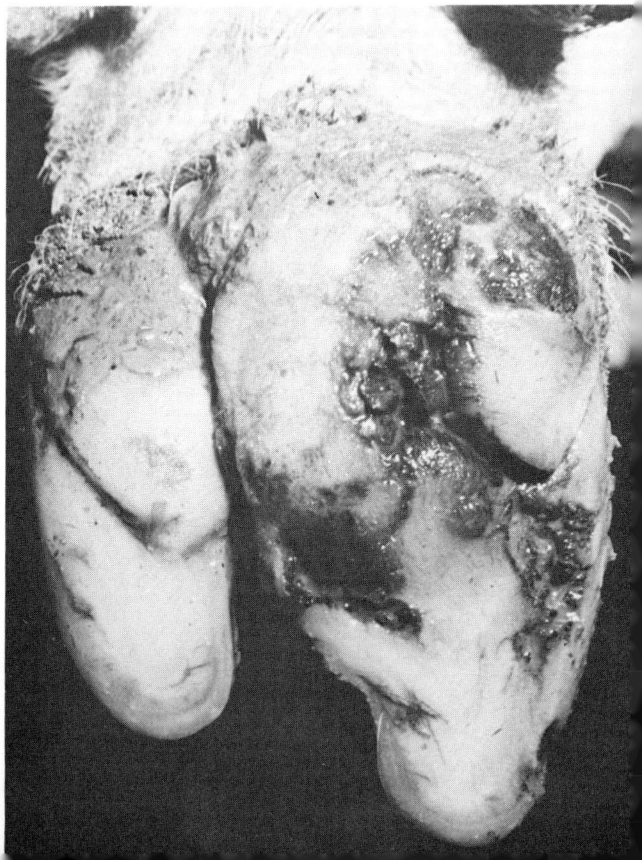

Bush foot, caused by floors that are not only rough but wet and dirty, is sufficiently painful to put a pig off its feed.

Photos by Dr R. H. C. Penny

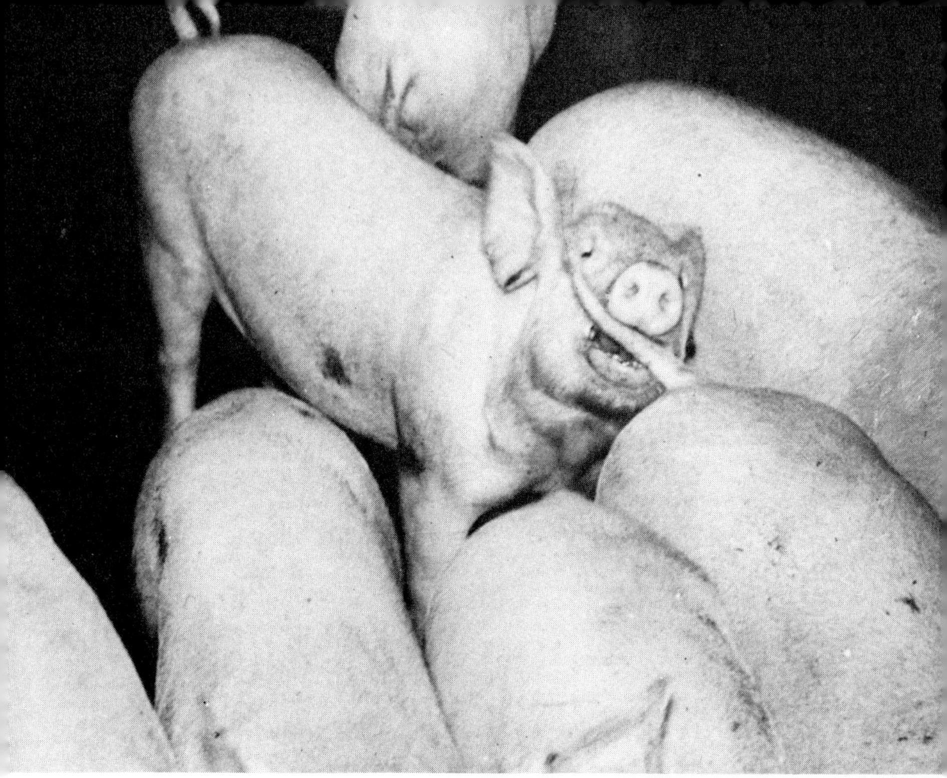

Tail-biting has become increasingly common among intensively-housed pigs.
Photo by J. N. Gadd

Stockholm tar is a useful remedy for tails that have been bitten.

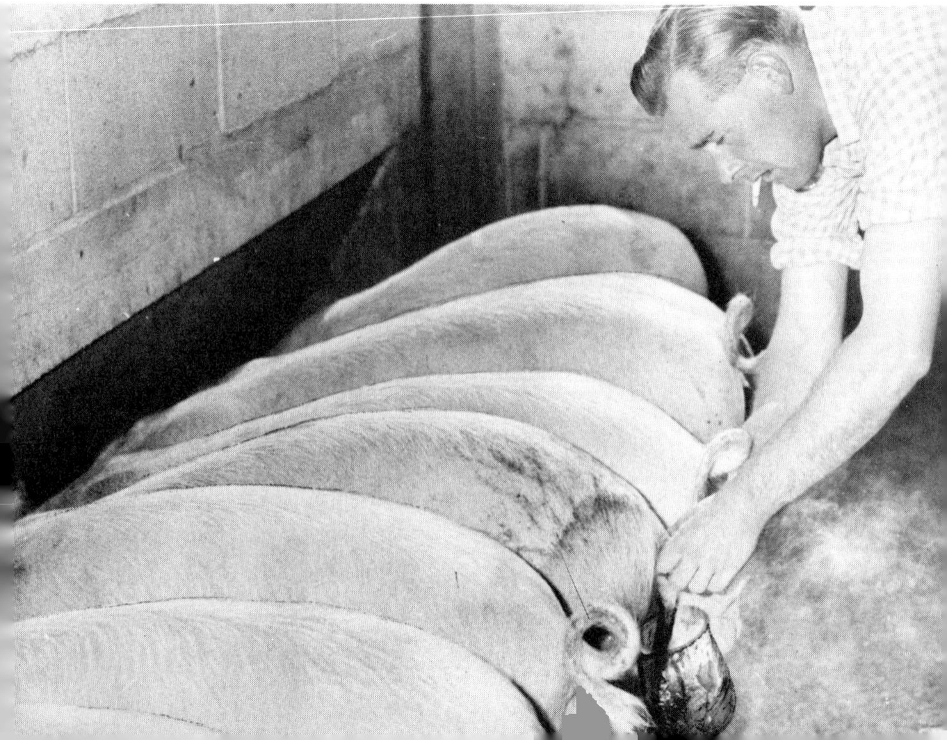

calculated to do almost as well and requiring less overall control. Crossbreds originating from hysterectomy-derived parents of selected blood lines are now available and can provide the basis of a high quality herd.

Atrophic Rhinitis

This is a disease which is widespread in America and in the Scandinavian countries. While it may have existed in this country for some time, it was certainly not a problem of any economic significance and received no attention until a flare-up occurred following the introduction to Great Britain of the Swedish Landrace breed. It has now become endemic in this country and is widespread. Because of the great variations of symptoms, diagnosis is very difficult in many cases, thus making it quite impracticable to schedule as a notifiable disease.

There appear to be two forms of this disease. The first is the so-called inclusion body rhinitis due to a virus. The virus is often generalised throughout the body. The disease is very widespread among herds, though it may pass unnoticed as it may assume a mild form. In the acute form, however, it is characterised by snuffling and a nasal discharge often containing blood.

The nasal region becomes swollen and there is much sneezing. The nose is obviously tender, for the piglet will not push its way among its mates in order to get food and in other ways it protects its snout from injury. It is disinclined to eat dry food and favours wet mash.

Breathing seems to be difficult and is obviously laboured at times, due to the nasal obstruction. The paper-like coils of thin bone that fill up the anterior part of the nose (the so-called turbinate bones) are red and swollen. The disease is progressive resulting subsequently in a twisting of the snout in an upwards or sideways direction. X-ray examination (as carried out in Norway and America) will reveal the extent of the damage and is probably a sound method of establishing a diagnosis.

The second type may also assume an acute or chronic form, but is associated with different types of bacteria. These cause similar though less marked changes in the nasal passages.

CONTROLLING THE DISEASE

Rhinitis is essentially a disease of the young pig up to six weeks of age, older animals becoming carriers. To control the disease, medication of food and water is valuable and should be introduced in anticipation if possible. This can be done from birth and at any suitable time. Management changes should not occur at the time medication is stopped. Reducing concentration of stock in weaner pools, so lowering stress, and not buying in gilts from doubtful sources are useful points to consider.

Swine Plague

This is the old name for what we now know as pasteurella pneumonia. The germ causing the disease is known as *pasteurella suiseptica*, and it may be present without causing harm. It may complicate an outbreak of enzootic pneumonia, causing more severe coughing in association with swelling of the lung glands and an increased congestion of the latter. It may also be responsible for an acute outbreak of pneumonia associated with severe respiratory distress. The appetite is lost. There is a marked temperature up to 105°F (40°C), the pig lies down as if exhausted and generally dies. Losses are usually heavy.

The more chronic case, which may be aggravated by lack of vitamin A, is accompanied by severe coughing which can either aggravate enzootic pneumonia or confuse the issue when a diagnosis is being made.

Affected animals should be removed to a cool, dark place and receive veterinary attention. There is a very good serum which will help to relieve the condition. But the best advice is to cut losses and slaughter out as soon as the disease is confirmed. The building should then be disinfected and rested for two weeks.

This disease runs a course very similar to swine influenza, though the latter is not considered to exist in this country.

Tuberculosis

Approximately 1 per cent of the pigs received for slaughter in the British Isles are affected with tuberculosis to a greater or lesser extent. All three types of the tuberculosis bacterium, namely, human, bovine and avian forms, may be encountered. In the pig it is the body glands and the bowels which are affected rather than the lungs. In the former abscesses occur associated with cheesey-like accretions. While the bovine and avian types are found in the glands of the throat with an occasional infection of the human type, the bowel and associated glands are generally attacked by the avian type.

Now that cattle in the United Kingdom are free from bovine tuberculosis, contact with them or the use of milk products will no longer be responsible for any cases. Many cases are, however, due to the avian type of germ contracted from wild birds or affected poultry, or through swill which contains the same and has not been adequately boiled. There have been cases of pigs contracting the human form when being fed on swill from sanatoria which has not been cooked.

Infection is seldom revealed during life and remains unsuspected until slaughter. Occasionally, however, more acute cases occur associated with ulceration of the bowels related to scouring, debility and anaemia, following on an early period of unthriftiness. Sometimes the carcase is totally condemned, but more often it is just the head and associated glands.

Some farmers go in for tuberculin testing of pig herds in the same way that cow herds are tested. However, this is not nearly such an important matter with pigs as it is with cows, except where the disease is persistent in the herd. As the main source of infection is now wild birds, control of the disease is somewhat difficult, as one cannot wire against their invasion. It has been shown that from 3 to 5 per cent of sparrows and starlings may be affected in some parts of the country. The highest incidence was in the region of poultry farms, but this is likely to fall now that systems of husbandry are changing—birds are kept more intensively and are killed much younger.

Tetanus or Lock-jaw

This condition is rarely met with in pigs. When it is, it is often associated with a wound which has become contaminated by earth. The condition may occur after castration or ringing.

A particular bacterium (*Cl. tetani*) in the soil produces a poison in the wound, especially in deep cuts which are not exposed to the air. This attacks the nervous system and makes the animal go into spasms of alternate stiffening and relaxing. Sometimes the animal remains stiff, the head and neck being stretched upwards and forwards and the ears firmly erected. All four legs are stiff, the tail is curled backwards and the eyeballs rotate.

Generally, only a single pig is affected and it is usually not worth while to attempt treatment. Where a valuable animal is involved, call in your veterinary surgeon who will probably be able to help.

Relaxation can be brought about by the subcutaneous injection of a 25 per cent solution of magnesium sulphate but the effect wears off after a few hours and the animal stiffens up again. The organism is sensitive to penicillin.

Swine Erysipelas

This disease is caused by *Erysipelothrix rhusiopathiae*, a bacterium which is capable of living an independent existence on the ground and outside the body of the pig.

The pig louse can contract the infection, but it has not been shown that these parasites play a part in its distribution.

The disease also affects sheep, turkeys and pigeons. It can cause erysipeloid in humans—a condition well-known in factories where pig products are handled. It takes the form of a painful skin pustule and inflammation may go up the arm as in blood poisoning. Fortunately, in humans, penicillin brings about a cure.

The disease is usually encountered in pigs in high condition, especially during hot, muggy, changeable weather. Pigs of all ages are susceptible, but outbreaks usually occur in animals of pork weight or heavier. However, young animals may be affected occasionally, even before weaning.

There is a loss in appetite, general depression (indicative of a high temperature), the skin coloration is often marked, and there is usually constipation. There may occasionally be very characteristic diamond markings or plaques on the skin.

In the less acute type, the animal may show vague symptoms of depression and may be extremely lame. There is often some patchy thickening of the skin, especially round the shoulders and along the back. Coarse areas can be felt adjacent to areas of normal soft skin. The surface is often crusty and irregular.

The more chronic type of erysipelas tends to affect the joints and make walking painful. One or more joints may be affected, and be hot and painful.

Post-mortem may reveal an inflammation of the bowels with a soft yellowish-grey deposit, together with some pinpoint discrete haemorrhages, especially in the kidneys. In old chronic cases, the characteristic cauliflower growths on the heart valves may be seen. These are caused by the erysipelas bacillus becoming caught up in fine abrasions on the flaps of the heart valves. Blood fibrin is subsequently deposited here and a soft cheesey growth builds up.

Sometimes the course of the disease is so swift that—apart from loss of appetite—none of the other indications appears. Indeed, a pig can be dead in less than 24 hours from the onset of the trouble.

Therefore it is wise to call immediate veterinary aid when a pig goes off food, especially when it is a bacon pig and when the weather is hot and changeable.

Penicillin is very effective and frequently employed. There is also a good serum which can be given as a curative. This serum should be given to the in-contact pigs as well as the infected ones, when an outbreak occurs.

Where this disease has become endemic on a farm, a sensible policy is to have all stock inoculated with vaccine shortly after weaning. It will give immunity up to bacon weight. In fact it will protect them for six months and, from then on, sows and boars should be re-vaccinated about every six months; the sows to be done when empty. This will not give adequate protection to the litter which will have to be done separately as indicated above.

Recovery from an attack of the disease gives a high degree of immunity, such animals being quite satisfactory to breed from in the future. In more chronic cases, however, the germ may establish itself in the joints and cause progressive arthritis resulting in increasing discomfort and difficulty in walking. Once the arthritic process has been started it may well continue to progress even when the germs have disappeared.

Wherever pigs are kept the organism of erysipelas will be present. To reduce its ravages to a minimum, however, efforts should be made to keep down flies, by spraying the piggery.

Swine Pox

This is known as one of the variola type of skin conditions which occur in all animals and humans. There are two types of virus responsible for two quite distinct conditions in the pig.

In type one, small blisters break out on the skin of the young pig and usually over the udder of the older animal. These appear as reddish circular areas of as much as one inch (25 mm) in diameter. In most cases only the spots and scabs are seen, and they will clear up without attention. The animals do not seem to be in any way ill or upset, although sometimes a sow will object if the udder blisters are rubbed or bruised.

The more serious and striking form commences with the appearance of pinpoint blisters distributed irregularly over the whole body. These may extend up to the size of a ten-penny piece and contain fluid. In a few days contamination occurs and a scab is formed.

Irritation is sometimes marked and scouring may intervene. Some pigs tend to become unthrifty for the time being, but deaths are rare and recovery is spontaneous in from three to four weeks. Skin infection can be spread by body lice.

The scabs, which frequently fall off, contain the virus and can persist for many months and be responsible for subsequent outbreaks. Isolation of patients and thorough disinfection after their recovery is therefore important. Lice should be destroyed and the skin sores dusted with 30 per cent sulphonilamide powder or an antiseptic dressing.

This condition should be carefully distinguished from non-specific eczema.

Heart Disease

By this is generally meant a condition which goes by the scientific name of *Verrucose endocarditis*.

It is almost invariably due to an earlier attack of erysipelas. In such cases the swine erysipelas bacteria have become established on the roughened heart valves and become surrounded by fibrin from the blood, as described previously.

The valves do not close firmly and the heart's action is impaired. Quite often large, fat sows which drop suddenly dead are found to have such a growth in their hearts.

The disease is generally not recognised before death but can be easily diagnosed at post-mortem.

In quite young unweaned pigs, it is common to find a large pale heart which may be associated with anaemia or possibly with a vitamin E deficiency (see under mulberry heart).

Meningitis

Inflammation of the brain membranes due to infection by Type 2 *Streptococcus suis* appears to be on the increase. It is thought that the bacterium spreads from the respiratory tract and from castration wounds. Mortality varies from 1–50% and death may be sudden. There is a high fever, reddened skin and nervous disturbance with blindness and deafness. Pigs lie on their sides and paddle and may show tetanic spasms. Some develop arthritis.

To control an outbreak, isolate all affected animals in a warm, well ventilated pen and give two injections of long-acting penicillin at an interval of three weeks. Sows may be carriers, so give penicillin treatment just before farrowing. In a self-contained herd the disease is self-limiting but depopulation is best with a fattening unit.

Chapter 10

SOME GENERAL DISORDERS

IN this chapter I will deal with some of the miscellaneous diseases and complaints that are likely to be encountered.

Sunburn

Young pigs under 16 weeks of age (especially of the white breeds) are most likely to be affected by sunburn and will generally recover when given adequate shade. Deaths are uncommon. Where pigs are provided with a mud wallow, sunburn is rare.

Burning of the skin may also occur if the creep lamps are hung too low in the farrowing house.

The symptoms are characteristic. White pigs first show a marked pinkness or redness of the skin, which later may become blistered. They move with a characteristic, uneasy, staggering action, frequently extending their legs and hollowing their backs as if stretching. There is a rise in temperature.

Affected pigs should be put in a cool shady place immediately. If unable to move, either rig up a temporary shelter over the animal or roll it on to a gate or hurdle and drag it to shelter.

Apply calamine lotion to the skin to counteract the effects of sunburn. Application of one per cent solution of picric acid may also be given (as for burns) but should the skin break, thiazamide cream is a valuable salve.

Use cold swabs—cloths dipped in cold water and lightly wrung out—to alleviate the distressed condition due to the heat of the sun. These swabs should be held against the back of the head (behind the crest of the skull and between the ears) and should be renewed as their coolness is reduced.

Electric Shock and Lightning Stroke

Where a pig has been subject to electric shock or lightning stroke the revealing factor will most likely be scorch marks on the body. Apart from these the animal may be dazed, comatose or dead.

If still alive and anywhere near bacon weight, it will probably be best to arrange for slaughter as soon as possible. There is a risk of the animal having suffered some internal injury which might also cause sudden death.

Where an attempt is to be made to nurse the affected animal, keep it warm—using sacks or rugs as necessary, rub any parts of the body that show signs of paralysis and call in your vet.

Heat Stroke

This must not be confused with sunstroke. It is due to the actual intensity of heat to which the pigs are exposed. The infra-red rays of the sun do the damage.

It may occur as a result of the direct action of the sun's rays on the pig's body during intensely hot weather. It may also occur indoors in badly-ventilated, overcrowded conditions.

There is great distress with breathlessness and a considerable rise in temperature. Sometimes frothy mucus drops from the nostrils and the mouth. The limbs tremble, there are convulsive movements and the animal may be unable to stand. Death may occur, but most animals recover if they are quickly moved to better conditions.

Provide shelter, soft bedding of hay or dried grass, and place wet sacks across the body. You can also apply cold swabs as suggested for sunstroke. This treatment will usually give relief if given early enough.

Heat stroke frequently occurs with fat pigs in show-yards or on a rail or road journey, especially after hot, humid nights. So be prepared for it in these circumstances.

Congenital Trembles

This is sometimes referred to as chorea or St. Vitus's Dance. In chapter 4 there is a list of conditions sometimes found in young pigs and believed to be inherited. "Trembling" is one of them. Piglets show signs of the affection when only a few days old and may not throw it off until nearly three months old. They bob their heads and jiggle their legs, but are otherwise healthy, eating and sleeping well. Recovery is generally spontaneous.

Before swine fever was brought under control 12-15 per cent of cases were thought to be due to the virus penetrating the foetus before birth. Brain and spinal lesions confirmed this.

Haematoma of the Ear

The long ears of pigs are liable to injury when violently flapped, when the pigs are caught by the ears, or involved in a struggle with other animals in confined quarters, or when they rub their ears violently because of irritation caused by mange, sunburn, etc. Blood may collect between the layers of skin.

When this happens the ears should be cleansed with a mild cooling disinfectant such as surgical spirit and be punctured with a needle in a number of places to allow the fluid to pass gently away.

A more drastic, but probably more rapidly effective, method is to make a slit several inches long at the lowest part of the swelling on the inner side to permit complete evacuation of the contents. Then dust the inside of the cavity and the whole of the ear with sulphanilamide powder; lay cotton wool or tow on the inner side of the ear as a kind of support and bind it with a bandage.

It may be necessary to insert a number of stitches through the ear to keep the flaps in place. This is an operation that is best left in the hands of a veterinary surgeon. If you make a long incision and evacuate the contents and do nothing more, further flapping will only encourage more bleeding.

Canker

Canker is due to an accumulation of grease and skin debris in the ear. It may, in itself, cause considerable irritation, but as the ear is frequently a reservoir of skin parasites, these may well aggravate the condition and necessitate attention. Clean the ears with swabs of tow or cotton wool on the end of a pair of forceps, or secure to the handle of a wooden spoon. Soak the swab in hot water, to which washing soda has been added, and finish off in clean water. When the ears are dry, dust with sulphanilamide powder or a borax-iodoform mixture.

Scouring (Diarrhoea)

The consistency of dung from a normal healthy animal may vary appreciably, according to the conditions under which it is being kept and the food it is being given. If, however, dunging is severe and the dung is more liquid than is generally consistent with health, the animal is described as suffering from scour. Such a contingency is associated with an inflammation of the bowel (enteritis) and/or inflammation of the stomach (gastritis).

Up to Three Days: Scouring at three days old is certainly not due to anaemia, but it may be caused by the sow's milk being too rich through her being wrongly fed or restricted in her water intake. It may also be due to an infection by *E. coli.* Many cases at this stage are however so acute that no scouring is seen—only a dead piglet! If there is time it is worth while giving the piglets sulphamezathine or a course of one of the antibiotics (see *E. coli* scours for further details). A brief scouring at three days may occur because the dam is on heat.

Some sows come into season at about three days after farrowing, when their milk is temporarily reduced. This seems to cause a digestive upset which, however, passes off after a few days. This is the stage to give the first treatment against anaemia. If scouring appears subsequently in the absence of anaemia treatment, then lack of iron is probably responsible or damp, draughty surroundings.

At Three Weeks of Age: At this stage scouring is frequently due to anaemia or piglets may be taking creep food which perhaps is too strong or contains too much fibre. Cold, damp, draughty conditions may prevail and be significant, as piglets are inclined at this age to stray from their creep.

Also, at this period many sows display signs of heat, again, when their milk appears temporarily to upset their piglets. If scouring at this stage is persistent, despite anti-anaemia treatment, call in your veterinary surgeon to apply treatment. Half an ounce (14 g) of yeast per piglet mixed in with the creep food is frequently beneficial.

At Weaning: Scours may be due to a too rapid changeover to growers' meal. This should be done gradually, mixing it in with the creep food starting several weeks before. The stress of removal to a weaner pool may also precipitate scours.

In Older Animals: Scouring in pigs of 14 weeks and over may be due to a variety of infectious conditions, all of which are referred to in this book—pneumonia, salmonella infections, swine fever, erysipelas, round worm infestation, swine dysentery, etc.

Dysentery and Other Forms of Bloody Scour

Faeces may be tinged brown by decomposing blood or there may be clear signs of fresh undecomposed blood. These circumstances suggest a number of possibilities such as:

1. Dysentery due to a sphirochaete—*Treponema hyodysenteriae.*
2. An attack of *hepatosis dietetica.*
3. The presence of *Balantidium coli.*
4. The effects of mouldy barley.
5. Niacin deficiency.
6. White pig disease (see Ulcers, page 98).

Differential diagnosis is sometimes difficult but often it will be possible to establish the presence of a condition now widely described as swine dysentery. To do this all the facts must be considered. A wide age range of pigs may be affected but it is those between 8 and 16 weeks old which appear most susceptible. Symptoms may be very mild in the majority of cases and death is the exception. In other instances mortality may reach 50 per cent. Traces of fresh blood or brownish-tinged dung are often observed. The greatest loss is caused by overall unthriftiness and delayed growth. At post-mortem gastritis is sometimes seen, but more often inflammation of the upper bowel.

Whilst the significance of various vibrios such as *Balantidium coli* and *V. duodenale* in bloody scours has been the cause of much debate, it now appears that the parasite most commonly responsible for symptoms is *Treponema hyodysenteriae.* All three agents may be present in the absence of symptoms but on other occasions their multiplication may be encouraged by the presence of worm infestations, acting as a trigger (see page 114). Average incubation period is 6-14 days, and the parasite survives for 24 hours at 40°F (4°C.)

TREATMENT AND CONTROL

While appetite is often suppressed, thirst may be exaggerated so it is better to medicate the water supply, though when it is necessary to add the supplement to the food arsenicals can be introduced to good effect. Too much, however, causes "jittery" pigs. There are now other good remedies.

An attack leaves no worthwhile immunity so every effort must be made to control spread by hygienic methods. The infection is spread in dung direct along passages or on boots. Once an outbreak occurs it should be isolated as far as possible. No fresh pigs should go into the house until this has been cleaned down and rested. A steady throughput of pigs especially from 8-20 weeks of age in a building without disinfection will tend to build up an enormous infection. Rats can be carriers and transmit infection to humans. It is always a good insurance to isolate incoming animals for at least a fortnight.

Transmissible (Infectious) Gastro-enteritis

Transmissible gastro-enteritis (TGE) was confirmed in 1957 in the UK and has appeared subsequently in sporadic outbreaks up to 1964 when it assumed serious proportions in East Anglia. Cases were also reported in other counties as far apart as Dorset and Yorkshire. Most of the outbreaks apart from those in East Anglia did appear to occur independently and were of unknown origin.

Many cases quickly assumed serious proportions, resembling very closely the disease as already known in the USA. These were marked by sudden onset and high mortality in baby pigs, reaching at times 100 per cent. This level declined rapidly to weaning age at eight weeks after which the death rate was low.

In young pigs the dung is a peculiar green colour, and thirst, depraved appetite and vomiting are common. Up to a week old, deaths occur in from 1 to 3 days after the onset of the disease. In older animals the picture has changed recently. Some cases now involve sows alone. They may show mild symptoms of scouring or none at all, and as not all animals will pass on immunity to their offspring there is often a recurrence in young pigs within a few months.

Post-mortem may reveal nothing, but in piglets, acute gastritis may be seen with ballooning of the bowels. The brain may be markedly congested.

Control. As the route of infection is either by inhalation or ingestion it is possible to get all breeding stock infected before farrowing by mixing fresh faeces from affected cases with the food. Faeces from young, affected piglets are the best source of the virus. Sows so treated become immune and pass on the immune bodies to their offspring and any other piglets which may be put to suckle them.

Injection of immune serum or antibiotics are ineffectual but feeding whole blood from immune sows is highly effective, the second dose of 10 c.c. being given three days after the first. The blood can be secured from recently-recovered sows. In an emergency it may be necessary to send a number of such sows for slaughter to secure 1½ gals (7 litres) of whole blood per sow. This is mixed with seven grams of sodium citrate and agitated to break down clots, then filtered and used or stored in a refrigerator till required. It is important to feed the whole blood for it seems that protection is probably due to the virus being neutralised in the bowel and, moreover, it appears that whole blood has additional benefits over the serum alone.

The most effective policy if the opportunity arises is to infect all pregnant sows not too near to farrowing by the method referred to above. However, it is now very clear that one of the commonest ways of spreading the disease is the lorry driver himself, carrying piglets and helping to unload or load them.

Much of the success achieved in the control and treatment of TGE is due to the pioneering efforts of Mr W. A. Noble, a veterinary surgeon in East Anglia.

E. Coli Infection

In recent years increasing emphasis has been laid on the importance of *E. coli* in the scour complex. Millions of *E. coli* are present in the gut, especially the large bowel, and are no doubt beneficial. There are different types within this large family, some of which have been found in small numbers in normal, non-scouring animals. Why then do they suddenly become dangerous and cause scouring? The answer is still incomplete but we have much useful information to help us in combating this problem.

Like ruminants and equines, pig-immune bodies are not transferred to the foetus but to the colostrum upon which the piglet has to depend. There are three such immune bodies (immunoglobulins) involved and present in the colostrum—IgA, IgG and IgM. Most of this passive immunity is acquired during the first few hours of life and is available for the first 5–10 days. But as the animal is unable to produce its own anti-bodies until about three weeks, there is clearly a dangerous gap here. It has been discovered, however, that immune bodies, IgA, can be produced by local stimulation of the cells lining the stomach and bowel wall. The material produced in the deeper layers is 'laid on' and protects the surface cells from bacterial activity.

This state of affairs can be brought about artificially by giving an oral vaccine in the food. Only so long as this is present will immune bodies be produced until the body takes over its own protection. Whilst milk is being taken from the dam, there is, however, some IgA being received but at a low level when the colostral period is over.

This form of vaccination is already giving promising results.

Each farm is said to have its own flora and therefore it is most important that breeding stock develop immunity to their surroundings. In self-contained herds this is automatic, but imported animals, especially if they do not go anywhere near the farrowing units or sow-yards, may farrow down and provide colostrum which conveys little or no protection to the piglets in this new environment. Death may then occur within a few days—even without scours—due to acute coliform infection, while litters born of indigenous mothers remain unaffected.

The difference in the pattern of scouring from farm to farm is due to (1) a variation in the degree of immunity passed on in the colostrum (2) to the degree of exposure of piglets to pathogenic types of *E. coli*. Exposure can be high, but because resistance is also high, scouring may be mild or absent. What we want to aim at is high resistance and low exposure.

We know from observation that immediately before farrowing there is a marked tendency for pathogenic types of *E. coli* to proliferate excessively as compared with other times. This rise in important coliforms more or less follows the lactation curve. So you see how vulnerable the piglets are and how much they rely on protection through their colostrum. If the pen is clean and comfortable the risk is greatly reduced, but if sows are run through a farrowing house without disinfection taking place *between* each sow, the build-up of pathogenic coli, may be enormous—enough to overcome any immunity achieved through colostrum.

Exposure of bought-in animals to the right flora before farrowing is a difficult matter to advise on, but running them for not less than a month in an old sow-yard could do the trick. Home-produced gilts should likewise be exposed. On the other hand a lot of worm eggs could be picked up unless a routine worming policy is carried out on the farm. A useful procedure at this stage is to supplement the dam's diet with sulphadimidine. It can be given to the animal before farrowing at the rate of 4 lb per ton (1·8 kg per tonne) of feed for ten days. This is regarded as a 'curative' remedy. It is unlikely to kill all the coliform organisms, but may well reduce the count to a low level at the time of farrowing. To control the levels of *E. coli* in the large gut either 1 per cent lactic acid or a culture of *bacillus acidophillus* is being used through the suckling and dry periods with some success.

So the lesson here is to encourage the build-up of immunity and adopt a routine of disinfection in the farrowing unit so that you do not expose susceptible litters to massive infection. See that bought-in animals are properly exposed, and ensure timely and adequate milk flow by proper feeding and management. When the piglets are weaned change the food gradually to a growers' ration, but continue to restrict their intake for several weeks. Scouring at this stage may well be due as much to a sudden change in food as to the withdrawal of milk which still may contain small amounts of antibodies. Turning piglets out onto grass is an excellent way of avoiding post-weaning scours and in any case is a good practice at this stage, for a few weeks.

Red Water

Sometimes the urine from pigs is coloured pink or deep red. This is due to blood pigment passing through the kidneys from the blood-stream and occurs when there has been a destruction of the blood cells, as a result of some infection or metabolic disturbance. Haemorrhages may occur in the bladder (cystitis) or urinary tubes, in which case the colour of the urine is due to whole blood which, as distinct from the pigment, will settle to the bottom of the urine if allowed to stand in a jar. The causes of the former condition are not generally known (with the exception of the 'yellows'), but good response is generally obtained from a dose of Epsom salts.

Haemorrhage in the bladder or urinary tubes is often due to an infection from the outer passages reaching the bladder. This is sometimes progressive resulting in the destruction of the kidney tissue which may be extensive before the animal dies. The urine contains pus associated with the germ, *C. pyogenes.*

Call in your veterinary surgeon as soon as any abnormality is observed. The introduction of early treatment has saved the lives of many pigs.

Fresh blood sometimes appears in the urine following service by a too vigorous boar.

Lameness

Lameness has already been mentioned as a symptom of certain diseases—joint-ill, rickets, erysipelas, etc. It will again be mentioned in reference to foot-and-mouth disease in chapter 12.

However, lameness does arise—apart from injury—from other causes; indeed it is commonly encountered in pigs.

Large sows in particular may suffer from sore feet if run for too long on rough ground or concrete. The soles become raw and tend to drop and the condition is often so painful that animals refuse to rise. (see also Biotin page 91).

Sows affected in this way get progressively worse after each farrowing and their breeding life often has to be prematurely ended by slaughter.

A condition resembling foot rot in sheep may sometimes be encountered, in which the whole sole appears to be under-run and rotting. In such cases the foot should be carefully and thoroughly pared, washed with soap and water, then treated with chloromycetin applied either in the form of a spray or brushed on. The hooves can be hardened in a footbath of 5 per cent copper sulphate.

Good flooring indoors—plus ample bedding—and frequent changing of paddocks to avoid rough, hard ground in a dry summer or frost in winter is the best way of preventing lameness from bad conditions underfoot.

Staphylococcal infection is sometimes encountered in gilts. The stifle and hock are most frequently affected, these joints being painful though usually not swollen. Post-mortem will reveal a little bloody mucus in the joint cavity, from which staphylococci can be isolated bacteriologically. This condition responds well to sulphamezathine.

In many cases of lameness there is also arthritis, the joint surfaces being eroded to a greater or lesser degree. Such cases do not respond so well to treatment. Unfortunately, this state of affairs is all too common following an attack of erysipelas, where the process appears to be progressive irrespective of any treatment applied.

When things get as bad as this, there is little you can do. It is best to cut your loss before matters get worse leaving you with a casualty on your hands.

The way to prevent such cases from happening is to avoid the conditions that cause them—those cold, damp conditions that are responsible for so many pig ailments.

Stiffness and difficult hind-leg movements are unusually common in the longer breeds of pig—especially the Landrace. Weakness in this region is very important, and care should be taken to diagnose the cause. Undoubtedly, in some instances, the problem is an hereditary one, but in other cases the length of the pig has subjected it to injury in the lumbar or kidney region so that animals may move as though in pain. Such damage may be caused by belabouring the pig over the loins with a stick, or by "chivvying" a batch of piglets through a creep or orifice which is too low, forcing them to bend their backs unduly and damaging the skin and bones. The number of times that injury is observed to the bones of the kidney region after slaughter is remarkable.

Finally, don't forget that crampiness and difficulty in walking is all too frequently a sign of rickets.

Leg Weakness

Mild distortion of the limbs has often been noticed and passed over as unimportant, except by the breeder who wishes to show animals and is anxious to create a good impression. He is moreover concerned lest the deformity—a "dished" foreleg or a twisted hind leg—is transmitted to the offspring. Great interest in these limb malformations has been aroused at MLC boar-testing stations since it was more important to ascertain the cause of their development and which, if any, were likely to be inherited.

Results to date suggest that this anxiety is unjustified, but that the leg weakness is a complex condition and associated with many factors. By examining tissues and using X-rays it was shown that there was a characteristic change in the epiphysis of the ulna joint. The long bone of each limb has a cap which is only held to the main shaft by a cartilaginous pad until the bone becomes calcified. This is what we mean by the epiphysis. Management associated with stress and any fluctuation in growth rate can affect the vascular structure here so resulting at times in this lower portion of the bone being separated by muscular tensions from the main bone.

When kept individually on concrete out of contact or sight of other boars, the risk of a breakdown appears to be increased. A soft earth exercising area with open sides so that other animals can be seen, or keeping two animals in a pen, serves to lower the tension and reduce the hazard. So far it has not been possible to implicate nutritional factors.

Skin Abscesses

Soft, cold swellings are often to be encountered under the skin of animals of all ages, but more especially in older animals. In the young animal the swellings are frequently associated with the joints and may be due to navel infection. In the older animal such swellings tend to be present on the shoulders and the thighs and buttocks—in fact at those points where injury is likely to occur.

Abscesses may be as large as a tennis ball but the general health of the animal does not seem to be affected in any way. When opened at the lowest point with a sharp knife a strong-smelling greenish pus can usually be removed. Local treatment is then all that is necessary.

The remedy is to avoid navel infection by providing clean bedding for the youngsters and to inspect pens and paddocks, where the older animals are being kept, for sharp concrete edges, nails and anything that may cause skin damage.

Vices

More as a result of bad management than natural disposition, animals sometimes develop bad habits.

Cannibalism: Reference has already been made to cannibalism and the tendency of some sows to savage their young. Cannibalism may be due to a sow being disturbed by outside influences or irritated by piglets' sharp teeth, which make her bad-tempered and spiteful. Once having killed one of her offspring, even accidentally, she may develop the habit of cannibalism.

Savaging may develop in adult pigs which are overcrowded, and kept under cold conditions with limited bedding.

This may be merely a matter of bullying, and in this context arrangements for individual feeding are most important, whether indoors or outside. A full belly leads to contentment.

Licking: Licking of the walls in search of some unknown, but desirable, factor may frequently develop. Mortar frequently appears to be attractive and some kinds of metals, especially those containing copper, have a strong attraction. This habit may be purely one of boredom and/or may occur when the water supply is short and the urine becomes concentrated and possibly more tasty, or it may be due to a frank lack of salt in the diet.

Soiling of Bedding: This often develops where pigs are not provided with adequate facilities, or where it is very much colder in the dung passage than in the pen. The dunging area should be defined in some way from the resting and exercise areas—by a ridge or wall, and be lighter than the latter.

Tail-biting: Nibbling or biting tails or ears may start as a harmless distraction but more often than not it leads to trouble. The sight of blood may stimulate the attacker or encourage other animals to join in. Resistance in self-defence may lead to fighting and possibly a dead pig, if the aggressor is determined. If the victim slips away and constantly eludes the attacker, the latter may feel appeased and settle down with a proprietory sense of dominance. On the other hand quick removal of the aggressor may ensure that no more trouble occurs.

The habit often develops as a result of overcrowding and boredom, or may be precipitated by fighting when different groups of pigs are mixed together. The loss of the ears and the tails may be due to frost-bite and is not uncommonly encouraged by early weaning on milk substitutes. Animals get themselves plastered and start licking and sucking each other. In cold weather smear the tails with vaseline for the first two weeks of life. The condition is becoming so widespread that cutting off the tails may have to be adopted as a routine, otherwise there may be considerable financial loss. Biting often results in infection and abscess formation along the back and more remote parts of the body.

Straw-eating: The habit of eating straw may develop in some piggeries to a marked degree. Again, it is usually associated with boredom rather than to any deficiency in the diet, although it may be that some diets do not provide sufficient bulk and are too finely ground and the animals do not feel satisfied. Limited straw-eating in pigs over 100 lb (45 kg) is not particularly harmful but it may be serious in younger animals. Barley straw seems more attractive than other varieties. Some roots or a little kale thrown into the pen daily helps to break this habit, as well as that of tail-biting.

Fighting: Fighting among pigs may lead to serious trouble resulting in lack of rest, retarded growth and sometimes serious injury or death. The causes are many and can be briefly enumerated as under:

1. Sheer boredom, in which case give roots and greenstuff at mid-day to provide interest.
2. A restricted diet.
3. Lack of sufficient trough space.
4. Cold sleeping quarters leading to local crowding.
5. The existence of anaemia.
6. The presence of internal parasites.
7. Mixing pigs: it is not common for fighting to break out where large pigs are mixed with small ones, nevertheless in practice it is often necessary to make up uniform groups. It is particularly important in these circumstances that the newly-constituted group should be in a pen which is not familiar to any of them. When mixing odd sows, let them run together loose in the yard before penning closely as a bunch. They will seldom fight if they are all on strange ground.

The following are the remedies suggested for preventing fighting:

(i) Sprinkle a little salt on the meal once daily for three days, although don't overdo this as salt may cause trouble, especially if water is restricted.

(ii) Hang a number of loose chains at intervals over the feeding trough and one or two suspended over the exercising part of the pen.

(iii) Offer diversion by throwing in some roots of mangolds, beetroot, turnips, kale, cabbage, etc, from time to time.

(iv) Mix the batches together and immediately run them through a weighing machine and soak them with disinfectant before putting them into their pen.

(v) Smear them with bits of kipper or spray them with a mixture of 1 oz (30 ml) of aniseed in one gallon (4·5 litres) of pig oil or liquid paraffin. By the time they have finished licking each other's skin they will be friends.

Where fighting has started adopt any of the above tactics and also throw into the pen a used paper food sack or two. In the course of tearing these to pieces they will forget their enmity. A white plastic ball or two, 8-10 in (200-250 mm) in diameter, can also create a desirable diversion.

If the pigs are actually overcrowded with lack of trough space on a restricted diet, and are cold and hungry, fighting is to be expected. Remedy these deficiences and next time fighting appears feed at once.

Behaviour studies suggest that vices tend to develop when the normal psychological pattern of the pig's life is upset by pen design, pen numbers, and his pen-mates' age, sex and temperament. Overcrowding and floor-feeding only aggravate this situation.

The use of the new tranquilliser azaperone is reported to be very effective in preventing trouble among pigs in large groups.

As the tail more often than not seems to be the first focus of attention, the habit of docking when a few days old is now common (see page 70).

Chapter 11

POISONING

SURPRISINGLY enough, pigs do not often suffer from poisoning. One would expect animals with such voracious appetites, liable to eat anything they come across, would frequently pick up dangerous materials, but in practice this does not seem to be so.

However, poisoning troubles do occasionally arise so it is well to know how to recognise the symptoms and what treatment, if any, to give.

Acorns

Acorns make a good food for pigs, but an overdose may set up gastro-enteritis and may cause abortion in pregnant animals. It is the bitter shells which are dangerous, due to their high tannic acid content. Normally pigs split and discard these, the only ill-effect being marked constipation with black, hard stools.

The antidote is to give an oily purgative, from 1 to 2 oz (30-60 ml) of castor oil or linseed oil depending on the size of the pig. Alternatively, offer linseed tea—linseed boiled in water for half an hour—with from ½-1½ oz (15-45 g) of sodium bicarbonate added. Again the dose should be varied according to size of pig.

Dried acorns can replace about 20 per cent of a meal mixture although they should not comprise more than 10 per cent of a sow's ration.

Ammonia

Ammonia gas is present in the air of all livestock buildings, being produced by bacterial and chemical breakdown in the dung and urine. Its intensity is a rough guide to the efficiency of cleanliness. At high levels it can cause a big increase in the frequency of coughing where animals are already affected and thus have an adverse effect on food consumption and daily liveweight gain. When the eyes of stockmen are affected the level of ammonia is undesirably high. This occurs when the concentration rises above 50 parts per million in the air.

Arsenic

Very small doses of arsenic have a stimulating effect upon growth, and because of this observation arsenical preparations have been included in small quantities in rations of both pigs and poultry from time to time.

Arsenilic acid is sometimes included in the ration to promote growth and to combat vibrionic dysentery. Though much lower levels are usual, when included at about 600 ppm symptoms sometimes take a month or more to develop. These take the form of a slow shaking of the head and a staring look in the eyes. Inco-ordination of both fore and hind legs rapidly follows and tremors of the head cease. Blindness develops and animals are soon unable to stand. The symptoms are well described as those of progressive alcoholism. The optic nerve is damaged.

Arsenic can be found in considerable quantities in the liver and kidney cortex. If the poison is removed symptoms rapidly regress and arsenic continues to be eliminated in the urine.

Barley

The cereals fed must be of good quality or indigestion and worse may occur, especially if there is extensive mouldiness. This may lead to a true toxaemia (mycotoxicosis). This is known to arise in association with certain moulds as a result of which the vitamin A in the ration can be destroyed. Barley is sometimes stored wet and allowed to heat up. If there is plenty of air then fermentation will take place. Such fermented grain can lead to scouring and symptoms of intoxication. Furthermore, rancidity may arise, thus tending to destroy the vitamin E as well leading to a condition of muscular dystrophy. If dried too rapidly at too high a temperature deterioration can also occur and may have adverse effects.

Bracken

Pigs of all ages are often run on bracken-infested land and come to no harm. It is, however, now known that bracken, when eaten, can destroy and prevent the absorption of vitamin B_1, so that symptoms may develop resembling a deficiency of this vitamin.

So long as the pigs have access to water and are given a few pounds of a normal cereal mixture, they come to no harm even on heavily-infested ground. They will eat the fronds, stems and roots seemingly without ill-effect. The roots, known as rhizomes, are three or four times more potent than the fronds.

Where scrub ground is being cleared and pigs are restricted to limited areas, little pigs often scavenge widely and do not suffer from ill-effects of eating bracken, but sows and older pigs, unless their ration is supplemented as mentioned, may develop a temperature, lose their appetite and even abort their piglets.

When considering the causes of full-time dead piglets and mummified foetuses, the long-term effects of previous exposure to bracken should not be overlooked.

Buttercup

When grazing runs short in times of drought, a sow may be forced to eat buttercup foliage. This can cause a soreness of the mouth, developing into blisters and ulcers. Another effect of buttercup poisoning is diarrhoea.

A pig so affected should be given its meal in warm water so that the meal makes a soothing gruel drink.

Good ley farming will help to eliminate buttercups. On permanent pasture spraying with selective weed killer is effective.

Castor Bean

Occasionally, castor beans are unintentionally incorporated

in feedingstuffs and may cause some trouble. Symptoms of internal pain due to inflammation of the bowel appear to be delayed for some hours in the pig, and poisoning is not so serious in this animal as in the cow, because the pig is able to vomit readily. Once having vomited and developed colicky pains a pig is unlikely to eat any more of the contaminated food. If poisoning is suspected encourage vomiting by giving an emetic and then some precipitated iron.

Coal-tar and Pitch

On occasion pigs may have access to tarred walls or floors, roofing material, and shards from clay pigeons, all of which may if licked cause poisoning (asphalt and bitumen, however, are apparently harmless).

There is loss of appetite, depression, weakness, jaundice and anaemia and, in the liver, similar changes occur as seen in *Hepatosis dietetica;* the two conditions, however, do not appear to be identical. Creosote could be similarly dangerous.

Copper

Following observations that rations containing copper were attractive to pigs, experiments were carried out to discover whether the inclusion of copper had any influence upon growth rate. Since this proved to be so, a considerable amount of work has been done in an effort to establish the correct levels of inclusion of copper. While the ceiling of toxicity may be very high in short-term feeding experiments, great care has to be taken to introduce a correct amount when a pig is likely to be fed from weaning to bacon weight.

Copper is a cumulative poison, storage taking place readily in the liver, which if too heavily loaded becomes hard and leathery. As the inclusion of copper in the diet is increased, there is a steadily increasing stimulus to growth and liver storage increases proportionally. However, above a level of approximately 180 parts of copper per million (180 grams per ton) storage levels increase out of all proportion, whereas the growth stimulus tends to decline.

As would be expected, blood copper levels rise when a supplemented diet is fed, but blood zinc levels also rise thus reducing the risk of parakeratosis. On the other hand, a mild degree of anaemia may develop.

A few cases of copper poisoning have been recorded where pigs have had access to verdigris—the green corrosion on copper—perhaps from the use of old copper utensils for boiling swill or containing it. If bluestone (copper sulphate), a material quite often used on farms, is left exposed, pigs may attempt to eat it and may suffer accordingly.

Because of the undoubted beneficial influence of copper in controlling non-specific forms of scouring, some farmers have been persuaded to include as much as 500 parts per million for short periods. At this level it may well be safe, the dung appearing black and hard, but it is not a wise policy, however, to include such a high level owing to the risk of the greatly increased storage rate, already referred to, and the risk of poisoning the pig as well as affecting the liver and kidneys.

Copper poisoning results in diarrhoea and sometimes vomiting. There is very often acute gastro-enteritis with the passage of blood, and evidence of jaundice as indicated by a yellow skin and membranes.

There is some risk of copper toxicity when pigs are held at temperatures well above standard ones, *i.e.* 78°F (25°C) and over.

Cotton Seed (Gossypol)

Cotton seed contains 0·5 per cent of an active principle known as gossypol, which at certain levels can cause illness and death. Evidence of poisoning is slow to develop, but there is muscular weakness, respiratory distress and generalised oedema of the tissues, especially the lungs. The heart, liver and kidneys also show signs of degeneration and, in some cases, pinpoint haemorrhages. There is no effective treatment.

Fodder-beet

It has been reported that, especially when badly stored, fodder-beet may be dangerous. This may be associated with the growth of green sprouts and the greening of the normally white skin which may be present.

The chief symptom is a copious, watery, odourless scour.

The animals are markedly more nervous than usual, active

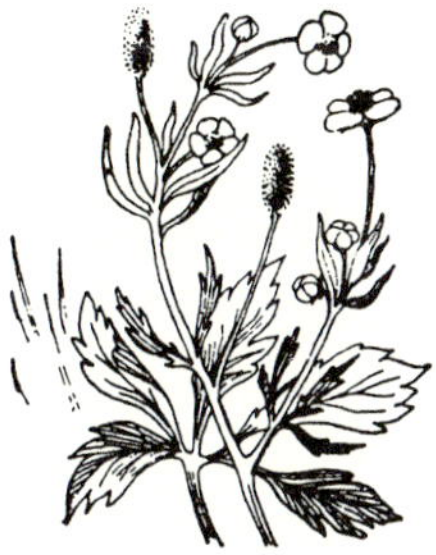

Buttercup

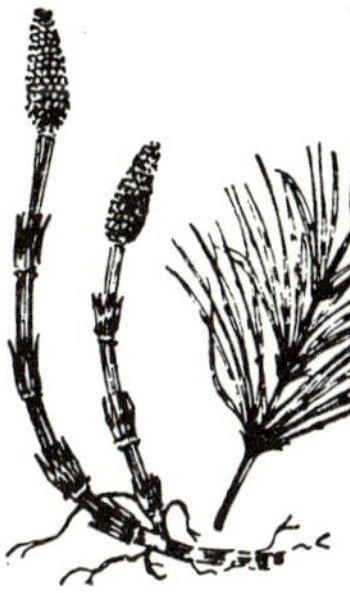

Horse-tail

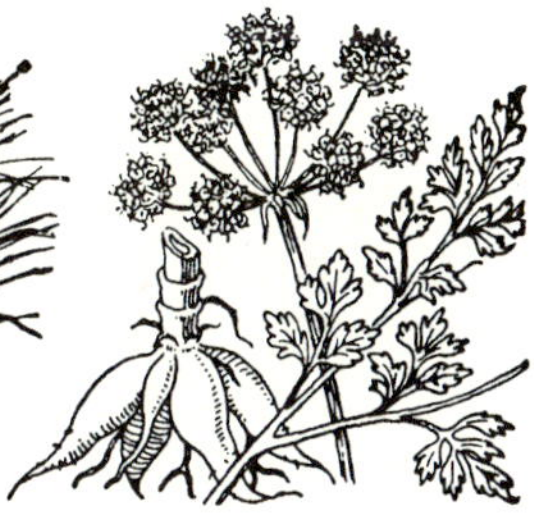

Water Dropwort

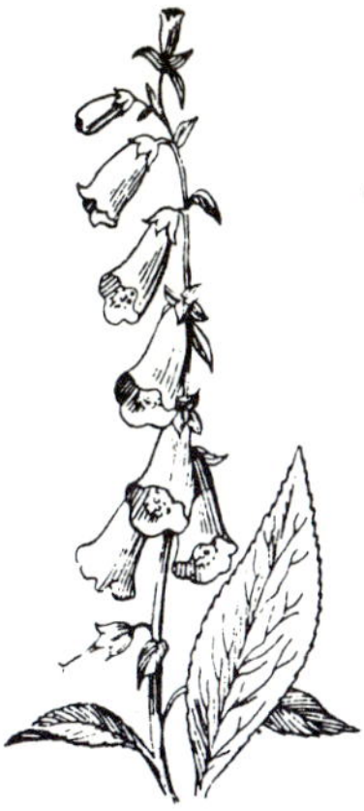

Foxglove

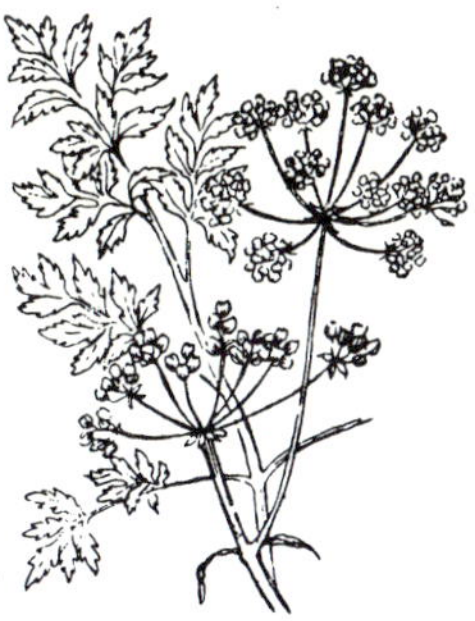

Hemlock

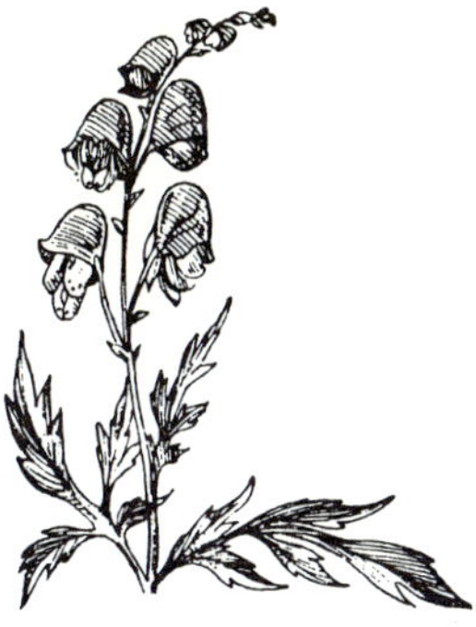

Monkshood

and alert. Appetite remains almost unimpaired and temperature is normal. The higher the dry-matter content of the beet, the greater the risk of a digestive upset occurring.

It is generally inadvisable to feed the fresh tops, unless the whole root is fed, on the assumption that the green parts may contain the poisonous factor. Frosted beet should not be fed. Two oz (60 ml) of Epsom salts ($\frac{1}{4}$-$\frac{1}{2}$ lb/113-227 g to the gallon, according to the size of the pig) would help to encourage bowel evacuation.

Foxglove

Poisoning from eating foxgloves is usually fatal. The poison—digitalis—affects the heart and, according to the amount taken, will cause excitement, quick respiration and heartbeats, possibly followed by coma, weaker heartbeats and death.

Give 15-30 grains of tannic acid.

Groundnut (Mycotoxicosis)

In 1960 a limited number of consignments of groundnut proved toxic to turkeys causing heavy mortality. The disease was described as turkey "X" disease.

After much research the cause was found to be a toxic substance (aflatoxin) produced by a fungus (*Aspergillus flavus*) parasitic on groundnut and other cereals.

The fungus has a wide distribution. It is found on groundnuts from many countries but rarely growing to such an extent as to produce dangerous quantities of toxin. The past sudden and severe outbreaks are difficult to explain, but the bitter experience has led to the elaboration of a specific fluorescent test which enables a working assessment to be made of the degree of contamination of a sample. Groundnut should always be suspect. Three-day-old ducklings are extremely susceptible to the toxin and are used as test animals.

Groundnut is a very good source of protein and is widely used. Though the pig is far less susceptible to aflatoxin poisoning than the turkey there is a greater risk in feeding young animals than older ones. In one experiment where toxic meal was fed on a restricted scale to pigs varying from 40-200 lb (18-90 kg), growth rate and food conversion levels were depressed. But there were no signs of toxicity.

Though diagnosis of the condition may not always be easy and some confusion could occur with other diseases, careful enquiry, supported by laboratory examination of the liver, should soon establish a diagnosis.

Hemlock

The symptoms of hemlock poisoning—either from fronds of

the plant or the parsnip-like roots—are salivation and inco-ordination of movement. An affected animal may have a drunken appearance. There may be convulsions and fits, and death may follow. Give 15-30 grains of tannic acid.

Horse-tail

This plant, with a preference for moist places, will upset pigs that eat it. The effect will be scouring and loss of condition.

Pigs believed to have eaten horse-tail should be given from 1-2 oz (30-60 ml) of castor oil or linseed oil followed by meal in the form of a sloppy drink. The weed can be got rid of by spraying.

Kale

Under conditions which are not yet clearly understood kale appears in certain areas and in certain seasons to contain a goitrogenic factor. This interferes with the uptake of iodine from the gut, so symptoms of a deficiency may appear.

It is thought that abortions and full-time dead piglets, may in some cases, be attributed to this cause.

Laburnum

The effect of eating laburnum leaves is nervous excitement possibly followed by convulsions, coma and death.

From 15-30 grains of tannic acid may be tried as an antidote.

Lead

As with all stock, pigs should be kept away from those waste dumps where old paint tins, tarpaulins and rubble, etc, are thrown. Otherwise there is a risk of lead poisoning.

Where the mineral naturally occurs in excessive quantities, *e.g.*, near lead mines, stock develop a natural tolerance to it and in such cases it is unwise to buy in pigs from other areas. Breed your own replacements or buy in locally.

In lead poisoning, animals may be found dead with—on white pigs—a marked skin discolouration of red and blue patches. Those alive show a lack of co-ordination in movement, leading to fits and paralysis. Abortion may occur in pregnant animals.

Where an affected pig will take food, Epsom salts ($\frac{1}{2}$ lb to the gallon—227 g to 4·5 litres) in water mixed with meal and three or four raw eggs is the best remedy you can try. Veterinary aid will be necessary for pigs that will not eat or drink.

Lime

A condition of lime burning sometimes occurs when animals are allowed to pass through gateways or over areas that have been heavily dressed with quicklime. The heat of the lime, following its contact with surface water or damp earth, is sufficient to cause scorching of the skin of the legs and belly and to produce a scalding or blistering of the parts affected; brown weals appear.

A similar condition has been encountered in pigs after being transported a long distance. In such circumstances a disinfectant or other irritant substance used for the purpose of cleansing the vehicle may have caused the trouble.

Wipe the affected parts with a damp cloth and treat the moist, burnt areas with boric acid, baby powder or a mixture of equal parts of bleaching powder and boric acid.

Mercury

Mercury poisoning is known to occur due to the inadvertent inclusion of dressed corn in the ration. Symptoms resemble swine fever and on post-mortem extensive haemorrhages are to be found under the skin and in many parts of the body.

Monkshood

Poisoning from this plant is usually fatal, death being due to asphyxia. In the early stages there may be salivation and staggering.

Try 15-30 grains of tannic acid.

Nightshades

All three types of nightshades—Black Nightshade, Deadly Nightshade and Woody Nightshade—are poisonous to pigs.

The poison affects the nerves and may lead to unconsciousness. Where dosing can be undertaken—*i.e.*, when an animal is conscious—give from 15-30 grains of tannic acid.

Oxalic Acid

Feeding of sugarbeet tops or fodder-beet tops may cause oxalic acid poisoning, especially if they are given fresh. Scouring would result in this case.

The tops should be allowed to wilt for three or four days before feeding; an additional safeguard is to sprinkle 2-2$\frac{1}{2}$ lb (0·90-1·20 kg) of chalk over each ton of tops before feeding. This is said to counteract any oxalic acid present.

Where oxalic acid poisoning has occurred stop feeding fresh tops immediately, dose the affected pigs with $\frac{1}{4}$-$\frac{1}{2}$ lb (113-227 g) Epsom salts and then re-introduce the tops gradually after taking the necessary precautions.

Prussic Acid or Hydrocyanic Acid

Pigs may suffer from this type of poisoning as a result of eating feedingstuffs contaminated with certain undesirable seeds. Java beans, for instance, occasionally get into imported feedingstuffs. The acid may be produced by linseed if this is steeped in warm water—instead of boiling water—for a few hours. When fed, the effect is immediate and dramatic.

Usually death occurs suddenly following violent respirations,

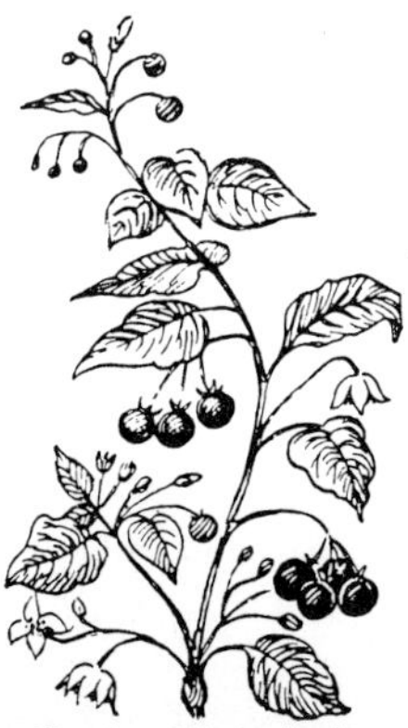
Garden Nightshade

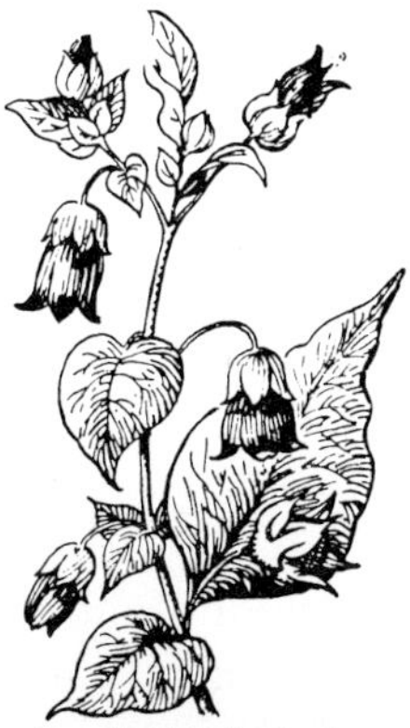
Deadly Nightshade

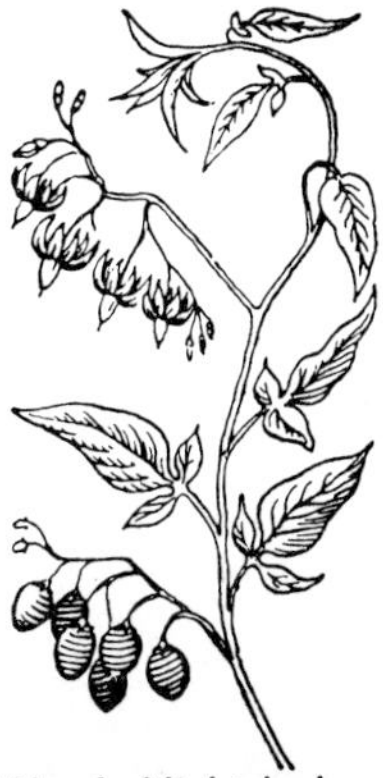
Woody Nightshade

salivation and vomiting. The acid paralyses the centres of respiration in the brain. On post-mortem a characteristic odour of bitter almonds can be detected from the stomach contents.

Rat Poison

A number of substances sometimes used for the destruction of rats and mice are liable to cause poisoning in pigs and should be treated with respect.

Warfarin is the most commonly used. There is loss of appetite and discolourisation of the flanks. Death is quite sudden. There is impaired blood clotting with cardial haemorrhages and pericardial damage, the heart itself showing remarkable resemblance to that of Mulberry Heart disease.

It is best to clear pigs out of the areas to be treated, to allow the process of eradication to go on unhampered for several days, later removing what is left of the baits before re-introducing pigs.

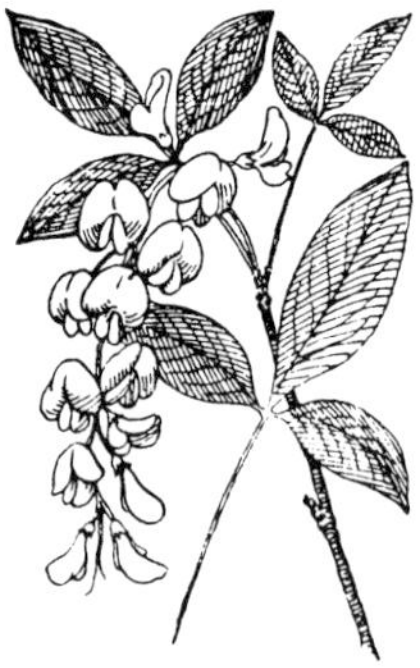
Laburnum

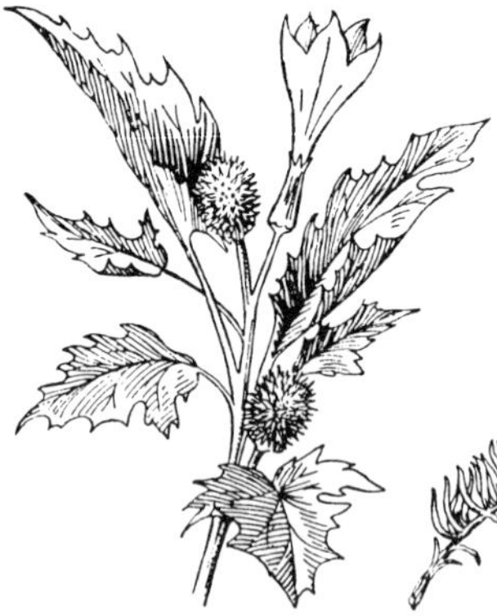
Thornapple

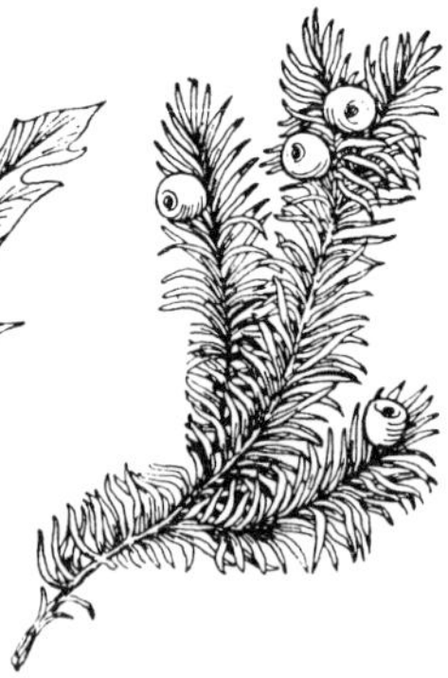
Yew

Rhododendron

Rhododendrons which are very common in certain areas, especially on acid soils, are said to contain poisonous factors which cause salivation, vomiting, abdominal pain, depression of respiration, weakness, staggering gait and collapse, but pigs, especially adults, appear to be highly resistant to their effects.

Salt

Salt or brine poisoning is probably more common than suspected and is apt to pass undiagnosed because pigs will cease to take the contaminated food and will then slowly recover. While it is recorded that no serious disturbances are likely if food containing up to 1 per cent is ingested by young pigs, older animals can take up to 5 per cent, but food becomes quickly unpalatable and pigs refuse rather than eat it.

Conflicting opinion as to the toxic dose is probably explained by the fact that while quite a small quantity will cause serious symptoms if included in a dry food, pigs will eat many times this amount contained in a wet mash with no apparent harm.

The usual story of salt-poisoning is that a number of animals are found dead without showing previous symptoms, the remainder of the group being weak and thirsty and passing copious urine. There may be violent nervous excitement, convulsions, then relaxation and a repetition soon after. Vomiting may occur. The animal sits in a dog-like position. Attacks become more frequent and end in death.

Salt poisoning may commonly arise in pigs receiving swill comprised largely of house scraps and pickled vegetables. Sodium carbonate (washing soda) may also find its way into the food by this route and cause similar symptoms. In such circumstances its presence may be masked by the prevailing flavour. There is some indication that brine is more potent than plain salt.

The trouble is often due to careless management and often occurs on Monday mornings, the water supply having been restricted over the weekend! Affected pigs should be given a plentiful supply of fresh, clean water and should be offered food in the form of a thin gruel.

Slurry Gas

Deaths due to continuous exposure to slurry gas have occasionally been reported. This misfortune occurs when a blockage has arisen and the slurry gas is unable to escape and rises within the piggery. It will particularly affect those pigs nearest to the exit of the slurry channel where the gases are most likely to accumulate under adverse circumstances.

Solanine

This poison is generated in sprouted and green potatoes. When these are fed raw there is a risk of acute poisoning. All ages of pigs are affected, the younger ones more particularly.

Symptoms are: loss of appetite, dullness, exhaustion, watery diarrhoea, low temperature and a comatose condition.

You can try giving from $\frac{1}{2}$-1 oz (15-30 ml) of tannic acid per pig together with linseed tea (made by boiling some linseed in water for half an hour) if the pigs will take food and drink. Otherwise there is nothing you can do for them.

Your main concern should be to see that the trouble does not arise. Potatoes should be boiled so that the solanine passes into the water and the water should be thrown away.

Thornapple

The foliage of this grassland (and arable) weed is harmless, but the seeds, when they fall to the ground, may be eaten by pigs and result in poisoning.

The symptoms are "gulpy" swallowing, drunken movements, depression, dilated pupils and rapid pulse followed by coma and death.

The best treatment to give is 15–30 grains tannic acid.

Water Dropwort

This is also a marsh-loving plant. It will cause diarrhoea, and may produce abdominal pains and convulsions. The roots resemble a bunch of parsnips and are more dangerous than the foliage. The antidote is the same as for horse-tail.

Yew

This tree, or rather its foliage, is well known for its fatal properties when eaten by stock. The berries appear harmless.

Pigs are as liable to suffer from it as cattle. The effect is usually sudden death although signs of excitement followed by coma may appear first.

There is no antidote.

Zinc

This is a rare type of poisoning and the toxic dose is probably very high.

When liquid foods, such as whey, are stored for some time in galvanised containers, there may be a reaction between the lactic acid and the zinc. This may be one source of poisoning; old battery plates and zinc-based paints are others.

Apparently this mineral will pass into the sow's milk and may cause poisoning in unweaned pigs.

The diagnosis is difficult as post-mortem will not reveal anything characteristic. An analysis of a portion of liver is the only way to confirm or refute a suspicion of zinc poisoning.

Chapter 12

NOTIFIABLE DISEASES

THERE are four diseases of pigs which need very special measures of control to prevent their spreading rapidly from farm to farm and so causing severe losses.

The law makes it an obligation for the farmer to maintain a record of all pig movements on and off the farm (including movements for service purposes) and to report a suspected outbreak of any of the diseases in question so that the necessary control steps can be taken by the police and the Animal Health Branch of the Ministry of Agriculture.

Therefore, the farmer's first action when he has reason to suspect a case or an outbreak of any of the following diseases is to ring up the local police station, explain his suspicion and then await a call from one of the Ministry's veterinary surgeons.

In the meantime, he can take certain precautionary measures to keep the suspected disease under control on his own farm.

Anthrax

As a rule not more than one or two animals suffer at a time from this fatal disease—and usually the older ones. Some cases may be traced to a particular batch or even one bag of imported feedingstuffs, especially when these are of animal origin. In other cases there may be a past history of the disease on the farm, or fertilisers of animal origin may have been applied within recent times.

All ages of animal can, however, be affected. In pigs the disease is less rapidly fatal than in cattle. The usual symptom in young pigs is a swollen throat, but sometimes there is nothing characteristic to go on and the animal may merely be found dead.

Loss of appetite, a slight rise in temperature, drop in milk yield in sows, signs of restlessness and constipation may be the only abnormalities. Unlike the cow, bloody discharges from the nose and anus are seldom present, but when an animal is suspected of having died from anthrax an attempt should be made to plug the orifices and so reduce the risk of germs getting on to the soil.

On no account cut the carcase. Handle it as little as possible and keep other stock away from the place where the animal died. Remember human beings can contract the disease even through small abrasions. Penicillin will bring about a cure.

Should a post-mortem be carried out on a case of anthrax, several feet of black congested intestines may be found, associated very often with widespread peritonitis and excess blood-stained abdominal fluid.

Foot-and-Mouth Disease

Like other cloven-hoofed animals, the pig is highly susceptible to this disease.

Lameness is common; in fact it may be the only symptom. The animal may show signs of considerable pain, squeal and move with marked reluctance. If on soft bedding, the pain may be disguised and the animal will try to conceal itself. On closer examination blisters may be seen near the claws, snout, udder or teats, but changes in the mouth are rarely observed.

The diseased animal often runs a fever and may quickly develop a temperature of 106°F (41°C), lose its appetite and scour or become constipated.

The virus which is the cause of the disease attacks various tissues, including that from which the horn grows. Once this is affected, soil and skin bacteria may become established and aggravate the condition. Claws often fall off.

There is no treatment allowed for foot-and-mouth disease. All infected and in-contact animals are usually slaughtered.

Should you suspect it on your farm, report your suspicions immediately, stop all movement of stock and do not go on to your neighbour's farm and do not ask him to come to yours.

If foot-and-mouth should be confirmed, you will receive full instructions from Ministry officials regarding the disinfection of farm premises and the lapse of time that is necessary before stock can again be kept on the farm.

Swine Fever

This disease, which is caused by a virus, is perhaps the best-known disease of pigs.

In many countries, though not now in the UK, the disease exists in a variety of forms, varying from the highly acute to the chronic type. The incubation period may be anything from three days to three weeks. Pigs of all ages are susceptible and if pigs of varying age are sick and dying, the disease should be suspected immediately.

The symptoms vary widely. There may be little more than listlessness, lack of appetite and "gummy" eyelids. In more severe cases there may be coughing, pneumonia, scouring or constipation, high temperature (up to 106°F/41°C) and sway-of the the hindquarters. Reddish spots may appear all over the body. In-pig sows may abort.

The skin of white animals may be highly coloured, though this is not a reliable symptom as skin coloration may be exaggerated even if pigs are suffering from a mild disturbance such as chill or indigestion. Diagnosis is therefore made more difficult. In fact, healthy-looking pigs can have the disease and be running a high temperature, whereas pigs showing the obvious symptoms may have only slight temperatures. In store pigs death may occur within three days of symptoms having been noticed.

Post-mortem is usually, but by no means always, a valuable aid to diagnosis. In a typical case, an ulcerated condition of the large bowel is observed and there may be blood splashings in various parts of the body which are characteristic. The history of the case is often more convincing.

This information does not apply to African swine fever which is a very acute disease with almost 100 per cent mortality. So far this disease has not appeared in the UK, but if it were to do so the consequences could be very serious indeed.

ERADICATION OF SWINE FEVER

When the disease is suspected control measures are put in the hands of the Ministry's veterinary services and appropriate steps taken to prevent spread. In March, 1963, however, an eradication and compensation policy was officially introduced, and the former use of crystal violet vaccine was banned. Though the need for eradication had been evident for long enough, the difficulties of quick and accurate diagnosis had proved a handicap. Now these have been largely overcome.

Full compensation is paid for all healthy animals existing at the time of slaughter, half for sick animals and none for dead ones.

The decline in swine fever in the UK since the eradication scheme was introduced has surprised even the Animal Health Division of the Ministry of Agriculture. Its success is, however, very largely due to the plans this department made and to the measures subsequently taken.

Many features of the campaign were to be expected from experience gained in similar ventures, particularly the quick disappearance of classical cases diagnosable by clinical features and the subsequently quick rise in cases needing more detailed and exacting laboratory tests for confirmation.

Swine Vesicular Disease

This disease is known to occur in widely diverse parts of the world such as Hong Kong, Italy, Holland, etc. The first case in England occurred in December, 1972 and is thought to have been introduced in meat that had passed through a middle European country.

The causal virus is of the entero-virus type, similar to that of foot-and-mouth disease, and produces symptoms which only an experienced person can distinguish from the latter. There are fortunately differences which assist diagnosis in the field. Only pigs are affected and tissue changes are not quite so severe and are more restricted. Lameness is not noticed unless pigs are forced to walk on a hard surface. The sores heal quickly and it is possible for a mild attack to pass undiagnosed in a batch of pigs on straw. There is a low mortality.

Spread is by contact with infected animals, premises or food. The virus is *not* airborne as in foot-and-mouth. It is tough, surviving 7–10 days in nasal discharge, 6–12 days in faeces and somewhat longer in slurry. The pig clears itself of virus in 21 days following the appearance of symptoms.

It is stable over a wide pH range and needs a strong disinfectant to kill it, such as an alkali (sodium hydroxide) at a pH of 12·9, or washing soda together with a detergent. Sulphuric acid, phosphoric acid and hydrochloric acid are effective in that order. It is killed by heat at 60°F (15°C) for five minutes.

On suspicion of an outbreak it must be reported; restriction of movement is immediately put on the farm only, with patrols established within a half-mile radius.

Restocking should not take place for at least 16 weeks and then only at 10 per cent of proposed full capacity, for the first fortnight. Any lorries involved should be disinfected with an iodophor/phosphoric acid/detergent mixture.

Swill is such an easy way of distributing swine vesicular disease and foot-and-mouth, not to mention Newcastle Disease of poultry, that regulations are at last being drastically tightened up.

APPENDIX I

THE VETERINARY CUPBOARD

Instruments

Clinical thermometer
Pair of 8″ (200 mm) stout, rounded-end scissors
Two pairs 6″ (150 mm) forceps
20 c.c. plastic syringe
Enema pump
Milk fever outfit (as used for cows)
Castration knife
Dog claw clippers
Ringing punch (for sow rings)
Wooden mouth-gag
Funnel and hose, or long-necked bottle and old rubber milking liner (for drenching)
Plough line (for restraint)
Wooden spatula or spoon (12″—300 mm—long)

Dressings

Several rolls absorbent cotton wool
One roll tow
Half-a-dozen tins antiphlogistine
Surgical spirit—1 pint (0·57 litres)
Calamine lotion—8 oz (240 ml)
Picric acid solution—2 oz (60 ml) (keep wet)
Pig oil—1 pint (0·57 litres)

Drenches and Medicines

Cod-liver oil
Molasses
Universal worming compound
Calcium borogluconate solution
Ammonium acetate solution
Ferrous sulphate
Copper sulphate
Supply of vitamin D—high level for supplementary feeding
Potassium iodide
Epsom salts
Linseed oil
Bismuth carbonate (or sodium bicarbonate)
Antiseptic pessaries
Dried bakers' or brewers' yeast
Penicillin cream
Sulphadimidine liquid
Sulphamezathine powder
Bifuran
Tylan

Disinfectants and Insecticides

Carbolic soap
Crude disinfectant
Mange dressing
Iodophor disinfectant
Washing soda

Discuss your cupboard with your veterinary surgeon and ask his advice as to what he thinks you need. Ask him to supply you with what he can.

N.B.—When measuring liquids:
1 pint equals 0·57 litres
1 part per million equals 1 gram per ton
30 ml equals 1 ounce

APPENDIX II

SUGGESTED TARGETS

No. of litters per sow during live time	8
No. of litters per annum	2·1
Age of gilt at farrowing	10 months
Age of boar at first mating	7 months
Conception rate: Natural (%)	90·0
Conception rate: AI (%)	80·0
Working life of a boar	2 years
No. of piglets born per sow	12·1
No. of piglets weaned per sow	11
No. of piglets born per gilt	10·9
No. of piglets weaned per gilt	9
Average birth weight per piglet sow or gilt	3 lb (1·36 kg)
Average weight at 8 weeks	45 lb (20 kg)
Days to bacon weight	175
Efficiency of food conversion (40–200 lb) (18–90 kg)	3·0
Length of carcase	810 mm
Back-fat minimum: loin	25–30 mm
Back-fat minimum: shoulder	45–50 mm
Eye-muscle area	27–28 mm

Environmental Requirements of the Pig

Temperature:	°F	°C
Farrowing house: sow	60–70	15–20
min.	50	10
creep	70–80	21–27
weaners (8 weeks)	65–75	18–24
growers, porkers (up to 120 lb)	62–65	17–18
baconers (over 120 lb)	60–65	15–18
heavy hogs	55–60	12–16

Humidity:

Relative humidity should not exceed 80–85%.
For every type of pig, the acceptable minimum is 40%.

Ventilation:

Farrowing houses:
250 cu ft per minute (cfm) or 20 air changes.
Winter rate: 25 cu ft per minute.
Production houses:
Summer: ½ cfm (0·007 m³/min) per lb bodyweight, or
40 cfm (1·12 m³/min) for porkers
100 cfm (1·4 m³/min) for baconers
120 cfm (1·7 m³/min) for heavies
Winter: reduce to one-fifth

Space Requirement: **Farrowing Pen:**	*Square feet*	*Square metres*
Sleeping and feeding area (including creep)	40–60	3·7–5·6
Dunging area	30–40	2·8–3·7
Creep	2 sq ft per pig, but minimum 20 sq ft with a minimum length 5 ft and depth 3 ft	
Total area:	80–100	7·4–9·3

Production Piggeries:	*sq ft*	*sq m*
Sleeping and feeding area:		
weaners	2·5	0·23
growers (or porkers) 120 lb liveweight	3–3·5	0·30–0·33
baconers	3·5–5	0·33–0·46
heavy hogs	5–7	0·46–0·65

Dunging Area:	*solid*		*slatted*	
	sq ft	*sq m*	*sq ft*	*sq m*
growers, porkers	1–2·5	0·09–0·23	¾–1	0·075–0·09
baconers	2–3	0·19–0·30	1–1.5	0·09 –0·14
heavy hogs	3–4	0·30–0·37	1·5–2	0·14 –0·19

Trough Space:	*inches*	*centimetres*
weaners	6	15·2
growers, porkers	10	25·4
baconers	12	30·5
heavy hogs	14	35·6
sows, boars	18	45·7

APPENDIX IV

Table for Converting British and Metric Measurements

BRITISH TO METRIC		METRIC TO BRITISH	
LENGTH			
1 inch (in)	= 2·54 cm or 25·4 mm	1 millimetre (mm)	= 0·0394 in
1 foot (ft)	= 0·30 m	1 centimetre (cm)	= 0·394 in
1 yard (yd)	= 0·91 m	1 metre (m)	= 1·09 yd
1 mile	= 1·61 km	1 kilometre (km)	= 0·621 miles

Conversion Factors

inches to cm	× 2·54	centimetres to in	× 0·394
or mm	× 25·4	millimetres to in	× 0·0394
feet to m	× 0·305	metres to ft	× 3·28
yards to m	× 0·914	metres to yd	× 1·09
miles to km	× 1·61	kilometres to miles	× 0·621

AREA

1 sq. inch (in^2)	= 6·45 cm^2	1 sq. centimetre (cm^2)	= 0·16 in^2
1 sq. foot (ft^2)	= 0·093 m^2	1 sq. metre (m^2)	= 1·20 yd^2
1 sq. yard (yd^2)	= 0·836 m^2	1 sq. metre (m^2)	= 10·8 ft^2
1 acre (ac)	= 4047 m^2 or 0·405 ha	1 hectare (ha)	= 2·47 ac

Conversion Factors

sq. feet to m^2	× 0·093	sq. metres to ft^2	× 10·8
sq. yards to m^2	× 0·836	sq. metres to yd^2	× 1·20
acres to ha	× 0·405	hectares to ac	× 2·47

VOLUME (LIQUID)

1 fluid ounce (1 fl oz) (0·05 pint)	= 30 ml	100 millilitres (ml or cc)	= 0·176 pints
1 pint	= 0·586 litres	1 litre	= 1·76 pints
1 gallon (gal)	= 4·55 litres	1 kilolitre (1000 litres)	= 220 gal

Conversion Factors

pints to litres	× 0·568	litre to pints	× 1·76
gallons to litres	× 4·55	litres to gallons	× 0·220

WEIGHT

1 ounce (oz)	= 28·3 g	1 gram (g)	= 0·53 oz
1 pound (lb)	= 454 g or 0·454 kg	100 grams	= 3·53 oz
		1 kilogram (kg)	= 2·20 lb
1 hundredweight (cwt)	= 50·8 kg	1 tonne (t)	= 2204 lb or 0·984 ton
1 ton	= 1016 kg or 1·016 t		

Conversion Factors

ounces to g	× 28·3	grams to oz	× 0·0353
pounds to g	× 454	grams to lb	× 0·00220
pounds to kg	× 0·454	kilograms to lb	× 2·20
hundredweights to kg	× 50·8	kilograms to cwt	× 0·020
hundredweights to t	× 0·0508	tonnes to tons	× 0·984
tons to kg	× 1016·0		
tons to t	× 1·016		

INDEX